Arranging Your Life

When Dialysis Comes Home

"The Underwear Factor"

Linda Gromko, MD
& Jane McClure, Interior Designer

Illustrations by Jane McClure

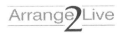

ISBN 978-0-615-32528-6

Library of Congress Control Number: 2009910000

Linda Gromko, MD and Jane McClure, Interior Designer, founded
Arrange2Live to improve the livability of patients on dialysis as well as
other chronic conditions requiring home health management.
They may be reached at:

www.Arrange2Live.com

Mailing Address:
Arrange2Live
16025 11th Avenue NE
Seattle, Washington 98155
Fax: (206)281-5088

Note: the above contact information applies to matters of Arrange2Live only.
Please do not contact Dr. Gromko at the above address for medical advice or
for matters pertaining to your own medical care. Thank you.

Back cover photo of Linda Gromko, MD taken by Cameron Karsten
Back cover photo of Jane McClure taken by Mickey Mansell

Dedication

To my husband, Stephen Martin Williams, whose journey through the world of End Stage Renal Disease and Home Dialysis highlighted the need for a roadmap to help others along the same path. I honor his bright spirit and his unquestionable resilience.

—Linda Gromko, MD

For my mother, Norma Johnson Chapman, and her mother, Veta Johnson, whose "skimpies," scrounging, and salvaging were the creative seeds that grew into my recycle, repurpose, and reuse. I learned from the masters.

—Jane Chapman McClure

Special Thanks to Our Editor

Our most sincere gratitude is extended to our editor, Jana Sawyer Prewitt. Jana's deep understanding of our project and her deft touch added just the right insight and refinement to our book. Her contributions have been invaluable.

Linda Gromko, MD
Jane McClure

Disclaimer

Arranging Your Life When Dialysis Comes Home: "The Underwear Factor" deals with the topic of kidney failure (aka renal failure, End Stage Renal Disease, or Stage V Chronic Kidney Disease). While this book does contain medical information, it is not intended as a medical treatment guide. Our focus is to help people arrange their lives and surroundings so they can live as well as *possible* with this disease—not allowing the disease or its treatment to consume their lives.

This book looks at the use of renal dialysis—kidney machine treatments—in the home. Making your life easier while on dialysis is our goal. We have had the most personal experience with *Home Hemodialysis,* using the NxStage machine. But we have included information on *Home Peritoneal Dialysis* as well. While dialysis methods vary, each method requires medical equipment and supplies, adequate storage, and a smooth system of organization.

Medical advice is well beyond the scope or intent of this book, and nothing in this book is intended to replace the personal medical information you receive from your own nephrologist or dialysis center. Please consult your own health care providers for advice on your care.

* * *

Jane McClure's illustrations in this book were done by hand to better demonstrate the "how-to" of crafting a floor plan. These drawings were originally done using the scale ¼" = 1'. During the course of scanning, and printing this book the scale has been modified.

Linda Gromko, MD
Jane McClure

Acknowledgments

We wish to extend our particular thanks to the following individuals and organizations who have participated in the development of this book. Some have shared specific skills and information; others have been there as sources of encouragement. We thank you all, and apologize to anyone who may have been inadvertently omitted.

We begin with the Northwest Kidney Centers and their Home Dialysis Training Unit. Most specifically, we thank the nurses who provide the one-on-one training and the middle-of-the-night troubleshooting. You are our lifelines. We recognize the administrative staff and board members for their tireless efforts on behalf of kidney patients in the Pacific Northwest.

We thank the staff at Queen Anne Medical Associates, PLLC, for their flexibility and moral support. You have been wonderful roommates during the creation of this project.

A special thanks is extended to Molly Williams Nyberg, who provided the CAD illustrations for furniture templates and our wall passthrough example, as well as useful suggestions regarding Ms. McClure's illustrations.

Our gratitude is extended to the following individuals:

Christina Anuntagune	Carole Pettes
Melinda Archide	Margaret Provenzano
Barbara Boni	Tami Pruner
Alice Chamberlin	Jane Pryor
Sonja Coffman	Sarah Rassa
Linda Franklin	Neves Rigodanzo-Massey
Teresa Graham	Lindy Russell
Brian Grev	Suzi Spinner
Carol Keenholts	Rex Stratton
Mary Ellen Maxell	Barbara Stratton
Donna Mitchell	Smiley Thakur, MD
Taryn Morris	Will Tinnesand
Gerry Morrison	Terri Weiss
Snow Nguyen	Carole Jo Williams
Janis Omri	Brita Williams
Bill Peckham	Bessie Young, MD

Contents

Introduction:

How this Book Came to Be

If you're reading this book, chances are your life has gone through some significant changes recently! You or someone you love has entered the world of kidney failure, dialysis, and now, Home Dialysis. That's a lot to go through, and this book is designed to offer some very practical assistance.

First, we'd like to introduce ourselves. Linda Gromko, MD, is a Board Certified Family Practice Physician and owner of Seattle's Queen Anne Medical Associates, PLLC—a small, independent family practice. She knew nothing about Home Dialysis—and little more about End Stage Renal Failure—until her husband, Steve Williams, tumbled headlong into Acute Renal Failure in September 2007.

Steve and Linda eagerly embraced Home Hemodialysis as a gift that could make their life better—but they soon realized that Home Dialysis brought challenges as well. Several months after starting Home Dialysis, Steve and Linda decided to try to sell their home. In the process of listing and showing the home, Steve and Linda nearly became unglued. How could they camouflage the dialysis equipment and supplies that had nearly taken over their home?

Jane McClure, Interior Designer and owner of Two the Nines Design, came to the rescue. In her work, Jane often "staged" homes for the real estate market: putting the finishing touches on homes to make them more appealing to potential buyers. Tasked with the project of staging Steve and Linda's home with all of its Home Dialysis accessories, Jane got more than she bargained for.

But in the process, Jane and Linda had the opportunity to learn volumes about the true impact of Home Dialysis on a family. Most importantly, they learned how to use a multitude of tricks of the designers' trade to make the process more livable.

The result is our book, divided into four sections:

Part One: The Basics

In this section, we tell you more about the story of Steve, Linda, and Jane—and their important realizations about making Home Dialysis a part of your life, and not its singular focus. We ask: "Why do Home Dialysis at all?" We discuss the two types of Home Dialysis: Hemodialysis and Peritoneal Dialysis. We look at whether or not a person is cut out to do dialysis at home. Then, we explore the basics of setting up your own "Home Dialysis Center."

Part Two: Bring In the Designer!

Does even the word "design" sound snooty, maybe out of reach? The truth of the matter is that *good design = effective function = easier living.* And a good designer knows how to work with a bare-bones budget. In Part Two, we explore how to use basic design principles: space planning, maximizing storage potential, and then the use of color, lighting, and furnishings to create a Home Dialysis Center that is both workable and comfortable for the dialysis patient and his/her helper—and the entire family! We get into nitty gritty detail, and introduce very specific suggestions that are proven to work. Best of all, we show you how to keep costs down and energy conservation up.

Part Three: All-Around Tricks for Living Better with Home Dialysis

In Part Three, we shift the focus to the caregiver. We recognize the impact that kidney disease can have on a family and look at specific ideas designed to help the helper. Most importantly, we look at how to prevent caregiver burnout that can throw a monkey wrench into the whole process. We look at ways other people can help, and get you ready for the lovingly-intended but rarely focused question, "Is there anything I can do?" We also take a look at reclaiming the bedroom and bath, part of staying healthy as a couple.

Part Four: Appendices

Here you will find even more specifics to help select products that work, find colors you love, and plan a Home Dialysis Center that really works for you. You will find lists of other resources that will help you as well.

Throughout the book, you will find real-life tips and pointers from the experts: Home Dialysis patients and their helpers, dialysis nurses, doctors and the like—people who have walked the walk and know what works. We call your attention to our website, www.Arrange2Live.com, for ongoing tips, products, books, and other helpful information.

Oh, yes—why "The Underwear Factor?"* Because Home Dialysis allows you the comfort of dialyzing in your boxers, briefs, bikinis or granny panties—dialysis *your way* in the comfort of your own home.

We welcome your comments and feedback. We wish you the very best on your important journey to comfort.

Here's hoping you all end up in the comfort of your underwear!

Linda Gromko, MD
Jane McClure, Interior Designer

* *Phrase coined by S. Smiley Thakur, MD (Steve's nephrologist)*

Part One:
The Basics

"Any activity becomes creative
When the doer cares about doing it right or better."

—John Updike

Chapter One:

The Story of Steve, Linda, and Jane

Although Steve and Linda had been aware of Steve's chronic diabetes and high blood pressure for many years, nothing could have prepared them for his precipitous free-fall into acute kidney failure. When Steve's creatinine (a kidney function test with a normal value of about one) shot up from an abnormally high level of four to an astonishing level of ten in only two weeks, the couple had very little time to get used to the idea of life-threatening kidney failure.

The stark reality was that if Steve did not receive kidney dialysis treatments (the kidney machine), he would most certainly die—in a period of one to two weeks! The other option, of course, was a kidney transplant—but that simply was not achievable in the short run.

Steve would require dialysis treatments three times per week. While each treatment took about four hours, Steve had to commute by ferry from his home on Bainbridge Island to Seattle's Northwest Kidney Centers. He could count on three full days every week—hours spent traveling to and from the center and receiving his treatments. While it would clearly save his life, Steve soon realized that dialysis could also consume it.

Steve and Linda seized the opportunity to learn to perform Home Dialysis. Home Dialysis would allow Steve to dialyze with

David Letterman in the background. It would allow him to stay more involved in the busy life of his teenaged daughter, Brita. In essence, Home Dialysis would allow the family to hold on to many of the things that End Stage Renal Disease threatened to take away.

(Note: for reasons specific to Steve's body, Steve's nephrologist recommended Hemodialysis. This type of dialysis involves the circulation of blood through a filter in the kidney machine, and then the return of blood back to the body. There is also another type of Home Dialysis: Peritoneal Dialysis. This method does not require the circulation of blood outside of the patient's body at all, and uses the patient's own peritoneal membrane—a membrane in the abdomen which coats the abdominal organs—as the filter. Peritoneal Dialysis is less complicated to learn and to perform. We talk more in Chapter Three about the two types of Home Dialysis. Because both types of dialysis require supplies and a system of effective operation, we believe that many of the concepts that help a person on Home Hemodialysis apply to Home Peritoneal Dialysis as well.)

So back to Steve and Linda: the Home Hemodialysis Program required four to six weeks of intensive one-on-one training—and the learning curve was steep. But Steve and Linda felt that the idea of Home Dialysis was a "no brainer." It afforded far more personal flexibility than in-center treatment. They also felt that home treatments might carry less risk of infection than in-center care. The shorter runs at home—done five days a week—were thought to offer gentler, more effective dialysis results. But most importantly, Home Dialysis avoided the sense of increasing disability which seemed inescapable with the in-center environment.

When they graduated from the training program, Steve and Linda moved their dialyzer—a NxStage machine—into their home.

Approximately the size of a small office copier, the machine sat on a portable cart and could nestle conveniently beside a bed or chair.

But then, the supplies arrived. There were sixty cardboard boxes of dialysis solution, each box measuring sixteen inches by twelve inches by eight inches. The footprint of the entire "wall of boxes" measured twelve feet by one-and-a-half-feet, and the conglomerate stood a full three-and-a-half feet tall. This represented sixty cubic feet. In a standard bedroom measuring ten feet by twelve feet, this volume would take up one *fifth* of the usable space! Taking up more space was a towering bookcase loaded with a variety of miscellaneous medical supplies: gauze pads, alcohol and iodine wipes, surgical masks, boxes of tape, IV solution, syringes, and needles.

Overtaken by the dialysis machine and its related supplies, the spacious master bedroom looked more like an Intensive Care Unit than a place to rest.

And if that wasn't enough, Steve and Linda were in the process of trying to sell their home. How could they possibly disguise this "elephant in the bedroom?"

That's were Interior Designer Jane McClure changed their lives. Tasked with the job of staging the home for sale, Jane got to work. With minimal time and expense, Jane re-created a beautiful bedroom—camouflaging the kidney machine and hiding its supplies while keeping the machine and supplies within easy reach for the near-daily treatments.

In the process, Steve and Linda made several important observations. They learned that:

- **Bringing medical equipment into the home— particularly an onslaught of medical equipment—can change the family dynamic. Rather than husband and wife, they felt like patient and health care provider.**

- Visible medical equipment says "disease is the theme of my life."

- Children—especially teenagers—may find the trappings of medical equipment frightening. Certainly, it can be something that makes them different from their peers. This can be embarrassing when you're thirteen.

- The idea of a bedroom as a place of intimacy evaporates, replaced by a high-tech sick room.

But after a simple, inexpensive "mini-makeover," Steve and Linda were able to reframe their view:

- Dialysis joins the family, but doesn't redefine it.

- Steve has a chronic medical condition that does require careful attention, but it doesn't have to overtake his life altogether.

- Teenaged Brita can bring her friends home without feeling self-conscious.

- The bedroom returns to its place of peace and rest, critical when life already feels like it is in the blender.

Discussing these concepts, it struck Steve and Linda how little they had thought—up front—about how they would incorporate dialysis into their home and into their lives. Sure, they knew how to perform a manual rinseback. And they could do a mean "snap-and-tap." (These terms will be familiar to those of you who do Hemodialysis treatments already.) But really planning for how this would work on a day-to-day basis? Thinking ahead about how it might impact them? Not a chance!

Linda remembers one time when Steve came home from the hospital after a mere three-day stay. An occupational therapist provided a raised toilet seat and asked if there were grab bars in the bathroom. Now that was planning! A light bulb went on. Bringing Steve home was like bringing a newborn baby home—planning, shopping and making some crucial changes would make it a whole lot easier.

When they brought their respective newborn babies home from the hospital, people gave Steve and Linda baby showers to make sure they'd have the necessary baby "stuff." Showers helped bridge the financial gap for all the things the new baby was going to need: furniture designed just for the baby, clothing, human waste receptacles, special lotions and creams, a place to lay the baby when it needed changing, warm comfortable blankets, clothing, diapers, CDs for auditory stimulation, safety-conscious high chairs and car seats, and the list went on and on.

Like most new parents, Steve and Linda also considered the "right" colors for baby nurseries, the proper ergonomic arrangements for caring for a newborn, and provided a comfortable rocking chair for mom to relax as she nursed. They even provided soothing music for the new baby. In other words, they *arranged their environment* to make the changes more comfortable—to make things work more smoothly. They *arranged their lives* to embrace the challenges ahead so that they could function as efficiently and as comfortably as possible each and every day.

The parallels in getting ready for a new baby and getting ready for Home Dialysis hit Linda like a ton of bricks. They really hadn't prepared much for bringing dialysis into their home at all. Why not?

For one thing, dialysis can be stressful—particularly if you don't have much warning. There is simply a lot to do, and the stakes for doing it correctly are high. Beyond this, the kidney patient may not feel well. At the very least, there are better days and worse days. And the routines of daily life—shopping, cooking, doing laundry, going to medical appointments—certainly don't stop when dialysis moves home.

As a result, planning for Home Dialysis can become an afterthought. It might even seem a frill. But, once we had the experience, we found planning to be more relevant and more important than we imagined.

Jane and Linda thought: what a wonderful service it would be if people who had already been down the road of Home Dialysis could help those who were just starting along its path.

Perhaps we could help people faced with the sobering realities of kidney failure:

- **Enjoy more functional, organized homes**
- **Relax in attractive bedrooms that invite rest and relief**
- **Create order when everything seems to be in chaos.**

Join us now as we walk through the process of *Arranging Your Life When Dialysis Comes Home.* We hope our useful ideas and strategies make your life better. We invite you to use our website, www.Arrange2Live.com, for more tricks of the trade, books, and products that can make your life with dialysis easier.

After all, as practical people, we recognize that illness is a fact of our lives. Living the best life possible—whatever the circumstances—is what this book is all about.

Chapter Two:

Why Do Home Dialysis Anyway?

It's a reasonable question: why do Home Dialysis at all when there are plenty of centers, both public and private, that can provide this service? All dialysis patients will experience their initial dialysis treatments in a hospital or in a center, and even Home Dialysis patients may have to go into the hospital or center from time to time. (Examples include technical difficulties that cannot be solved at home, the need for services such as blood transfusions which cannot be given at home, or the temporary illness or absence of the dialysis helper.)

Home Dialysis takes a special kind of effort on the part of everyone involved. So why do it?

Reason # 1: Comfort

Dr. Smiley Thakur, Steve's nephrologist, called it *"The Underwear Factor."* What he meant was that at home, you can dialyze in your boxer shorts if you want. You can spend time with your family. You can have friends over—at least the kind of friends who can watch your dialysis treatments in comfort. You can eat what you like, and watch TV with the volume up as loud as your spouse will tolerate. Basically, you are in your own home—and it feels good and normal to be there.

Reason # 2: Flexibility

Most dialysis centers give you an assigned schedule for Hemodialysis: four hour treatments done three times a week. You must dialyze when the center is open, and that's according to their schedule—not yours. Suppose you want to attend a family party or a nephew's graduation? What if you just want to sleep in one day, and do a treatment later in the evening? This is all possible when you set the schedule.

Reason # 3: Gentler, More Effective Dialysis

Doing dialysis at home allows you to do more frequent treatments, and often at a gentler pace. Many medical experts believe that more frequent treatments are more effective in mimicking natural kidney function. And why not? Normal kidneys are on the job 24/7. Gentler, more frequent dialysis also avoids wide swings in body fluid volume. People may not feel as "wrung out" as with three-day-a-week treatments. And you may have more flexibility with your diet—not having to be quite so restrictive in what you eat.

Reason # 4: Infection Control

It makes sense that if you do dialysis in your own home, you will be exposed to fewer colds, viral infections, and bacterial infections than if you are treated in a facility with many patients and many care providers. No matter how meticulous the care, there is simply more chance of picking up an infection that a kidney patient doesn't need.

Reason # 5: Quality Control

While we have observed only superlative care at the Northwest Kidney Centers, it makes intuitive sense that you could get a nurse or technician you don't get along with—or worse, isn't as careful about how they do their job as they should be. When a loved one performs dialysis, you know they care—really care—about the patient. Nobody cares more about the quality of your treatment than you or your partner. (And, for that matter, if you do Peritoneal Dialysis, you have the ultimate in quality control—doing the treatments yourself.)

Reason # 6: Feeling in Control

Kidney disease can feel like it takes a lot of your life away. But as much as you might want to, you can't ignore it; you have to deal with it or you will feel worse and have more complications. Home Dialysis places you in a position where you truly have the most control over the quality of your life.

Reason # 7: You can go on vacation!

While it takes some doing, you can take your Home Hemodialysis machine on the road. Steve and Linda flew to San Diego for a business convention only months after learning how to do Home Hemodialysis. Other people take their machines on cruise ships, or go camping in the RV. Of course, you can arrange for in-center treatments in many locations, but the ultimate in travel flexibility rests with doing your treatments yourself.

Peritoneal Dialysis is highly adaptable to travel. You don't even need to take a machine—just dialysis fluid and supplies.

We've devoted a chapter to travel logistics, beginning on Page 93.

Reason # 8: The Opportunity to Multi-task

With a little planning it's possible to get work done while doing Home Hemodialysis. Steve conducts conference calls with business associates. He also reads and watches movies. Many people work on their computers.

All of this—and more—is possible with Peritoneal Dialysis.

Reason #9: Time Together

Kidney failure is a life-threatening condition; thank heaven we have the medical miracle of life-saving dialysis! But when you've been faced with this diagnosis, life becomes a little more precious. It's good to have time to spend with your family—even if it's time "on the hose."

Reason # 10: A Room with a View

On Bainbridge Island, Steve and Linda can look out the front window and see deer or pheasant in the yard sometimes. Most Centers can't compete with that. But no matter what your view is, it's home and it's familiar.

Making the environment as cozy, convenient, attractive, and functional as possible will add to your quality of life in ways that can't be quantified.

Chapter Three:

What are the Types of Home Dialysis?

Kidneys are complicated organs located in the area of the small of the back. In normal circumstances, we each come with two kidneys. Unfortunately, most disease processes which impact the kidneys (like diabetes and high blood pressure) affect both kidneys equally. We know that a person with healthy kidneys can function perfectly well with only one kidney; that's why a healthy person can donate a kidney to another person for a kidney transplant.

We all know that kidneys make urine, filter and eliminate toxins from our bloodstream, and keep necessary chemicals in. They eliminate excess fluid from the body. Steve gained about forty pounds in a period of weeks as he spiraled into kidney failure. Kidneys make a hormone (EPO) which tells our bone marrow to make red blood cells and another hormone (renin) which regulates blood pressure. Kidneys also modify vitamin D into a mature form essential for building healthy bones.

As most kidney patients know, we can get EPO in an injectable form. And there are a number of ways to get additional vitamin D.

But when it comes to removing toxins and extra fluids from the body, you've got to have a kidney—or a dialysis process to do the work. Hemodialysis and Peritoneal Dialysis both rely on a filter to remove toxins and squeeze out the body's excess fluids.

Which dialysis option a patient uses may depend on personal preference—but there are also factors specific to each individual patient which may make one form of dialysis preferable over another. We'll leave that choice to the patient and his or her nephrologist. But here are the basics:

In **Hemodialysis**, blood is circulated outside of the patient's body to a dialysis machine. The blood is then circulated through a filter and returned to the body by way of plastic tubing. The blood leaves and enters the body through a specially created "access" location. This is either a temporary "central line"—a large IV portal in the patient's upper chest or neck, or a "fistula"—a surgically enlarged vein which is generally created in the arm. Whether using a temporary central line or a permanent fistula, there is an exit portal and an entry portal for the blood. In Hemodialysis, a patient must stay in the same location, generally in a dialysis recliner or in bed, for the duration of each treatment. Each patient's dialysis prescription varies. Many patients do three-to-four hour runs during the day, or extended overnight treatments during sleep. Treatments may be done three to five times per week, depending on the individual patient's prescription.

In **Peritoneal Dialysis**, blood doesn't leave the patient's body at all. Rather, this technique uses the body's own internal filter: the peritoneal membrane that lines the abdominal organs. In Peritoneal Dialysis, the access port is a flexible plastic tube which is surgically placed in the patient's abdomen in the neighborhood of the belly button. Dialysis solution can then run into the abdomen where it's said to "dwell," allowing the solution to interact with the patient's blood—with molecules wandering across the peritoneal membrane.

After the necessary exchange of molecules and fluid occurs, the toxins and excess fluids are removed from the body and into a waste bag or down the drain.

Within **Peritoneal Dialysis**, there are two variations:

- **Continuous Ambulatory Peritoneal Dialysis (CAPD)**—four exchanges per day. Before the patient's very first treatment, dialysis fluid is run into the abdomen, and allowed to dwell. The dwell time is when the exchange of molecules and fluids takes place. In each subsequent treatment, the patient begins by connecting the plastic tube to a set of two branching bags—one empty bag, and one bag full of fresh dialysis solution. The patient begins by emptying the dwell fluid from the abdomen—now waste—into the empty bag. Then, fresh dialysis solution runs into the patient's abdomen where it becomes the new dwell fluid, and another exchange process begins. Each treatment is done with new solution four times a day, but takes only about thirty minutes per treatment. Many patients take their dialysis solution to work and do a couple of exchanges in the workplace.

- **Continuous Cycling Peritoneal Dialysis (CCPD)**—Using a bedside machine to perform a series of empty/fill/ dwell cycles through the night during sleep.

In Peritoneal Dialysis, a patient must do either ambulatory or overnight treatments—or a combination of both—every single day to achieve maximal benefit.

Isn't dialysis ingenious? These techniques have saved millions of lives and can save your life or your loved one's! We all get it, of course, that there is nothing like a kidney.* Many of us pray for that transplanted kidney from a compassionate living donor or the gift of a cadaver kidney. But in the meantime, we have dialysis. And we can learn to perform it in the comfort of home.

---

* *Recent research suggests that frequent, extended treatments may be a reasonable alternative to transplant—providing nearly equivalent outcomes—for many patients.*

Chapter Four:

Are you Personally Cut Out to do Home Dialysis?

Home Dialysis is not for everybody. If you've already said "there is no way on earth I would ever do that," it's okay. Not all of us are interested in "The Underwear Factor". But if the reasons we've listed in Chapter Two spoke to you at all, read on!

In our opinion, *Home Hemodialysis* requires the following:

Requirement # 1: A Team that Works Well Together

Steve and Linda started out as a committed couple and actually got married shortly after completing their home training. Do they always work together smoothly? Of course not. But they do share a mutual commitment to doing the best dialysis treatments possible, with the intention of helping Steve live as long and as well as he can. They have established certain ground rules. For example, there's no arguing while on dialysis. It simply feels wrong—the patient is too vulnerable so it can feel threatening. When we describe a Team, we recognize that the dialysis helper might be a spouse or partner, a parent, a son or daughter, a niece or nephew, or a great friend. Certainly, if you have the resources, you could hire a trained technician or nurse. But no matter, you need a Team that will work together effectively.

Requirement # 2: The Ability to Read and Follow Directions

Following directions with consistency—even a bit of rigidity—is important. As Steve used to say, "Don't freelance here, Lindajo!" Following the rules diligently will keep you out of trouble most of the time.

Requirement # 3: Manual Dexterity and Physical Strength

Home Hemodialysis requires the ability to attach needles to syringes, draw up saline and Heparin into syringes, and connect plastic tubing together. It involves tearing tape to secure dialysis hoses, and the ability to firmly insert a "priming spike" into a liter of IV fluid. This might be impossible for a helper who has arthritic hands, for example.

Five or six five-liter bags have to be lifted overhead and onto the dialysis IV pole. Each bag weighs over ten pounds. In addition, cardboard boxes containing the five-liter bags of dialysis solution have to be opened, and the bags removed from their plastic outer-wraps.

One of our heroines is a Seattle woman who has performed Home Hemodialysis for her husband for many years. Both are in their eighties. She has a granddaughter who hangs the bags, but she glides through the rest of the tasks on her own.

Requirement # 4: Adequate Vision and Lighting

You must be able to see well enough to draw up medications with accuracy. Good lighting for this task is essential. Overhead lighting is designed to flood a room, but you will want a good floor lamp or task light with the capacity to focus direct light where it's needed to give you every advantage.

Requirement # 5: The Ability to Function Under Pressure

Everybody who does Hemodialysis treatments, whether at home or in a hospital or center, will sometimes experience alarms from the machine that may signal something is wrong. Some of the alarms are merely annoying, but others signal trouble that must be fixed immediately or serious complications may follow.

Training teaches how to manage these alarms. Alarms are signaled with a bell, and a visible number: yellow alerting us to a concern and red for deeper trouble. We learn to quickly look up the alarm number displayed on the front of the machine in our manual. The manual gives simple instructions for immediate troubleshooting.

There are two "hotlines" available for immediate telephone support: one from the nurses at the local dialysis center, and the other a technical support line from the company that makes the machines. Most of the time, you will be able to troubleshoot problems on your own. But now and then, you will likely call one of the 1-800 numbers.

(Linda remembers the hotline operator asking, "What state are you calling from?" Her answer: "From the state of confusion!")

If you know yourself well enough to know that you would panic under such pressure, this might not be the route for you. But truly, people of all backgrounds and abilities have mastered the skills of Home Hemodialysis. It is definitely learnable—and the backup support is extraordinary!

What about *Home Peritoneal Dialysis?*

In contrast to Home Hemodialysis, you can do your own Peritoneal Dialysis without assistance from another person. You must go to your dialysis center for training, but it's shorter: roughly a week as opposed to four to six weeks for Hemodialysis training. You, too, must be able to read, follow instructions, and troubleshoot—but the menu of potential problems is less complex. You must have the manual dexterity to connect the branching bags to your access port, or to connect your access to the overnight cycler. To minimize your risk of infection, you must observe good personal hygiene and proper "no-touch" technique. And, of course, you must have the discipline to "get in" all the treatments you need—and to do treatments every day.

Again, though, excellent backup exists in the form of your dialysis center staff. There are people who will lovingly guide you through the process and help you along the way.

Chapter Five:

Setting Up Your Own Home Dialysis Center

Steve and Linda joke that their home *is* the Bainbridge Island Hemodialysis Center! Perhaps there are others on our Island who quietly perform Home Dialysis—we just don't know who they are.

In any event, setting up your home for dialysis requires the following basic considerations. We'll go through each one before calling in the designer, and expand on some of the specifics in separate chapters later in this book. But start here for the very basics. (We'll address Hemodialysis first and discuss Peritoneal Dialysis at the end of this chapter.)

1: Where will you perform your Hemodialysis?

Unless you live in a studio apartment, there are several rooms where you might dialyze:

- **Family room**
- **Guest bedroom**
- **Master bedroom**
- **Study or den**
- **Dining Room**

We encourage you not to use your bedroom for dialysis unless you are going to do overnight dialysis in bed—and we'll discuss this in detail in Chapter 21. We show you how to use all the above rooms for dialysis in a way that is safe, convenient, and discreet when the treatment is not actively being performed.

Remember: unless you are doing extended runs and plan to dialyze in bed, a dialysis chair is required. This specially designed chair can assume a range of positions—including flat or tipped back to elevate the feet above the head, and ensures the greatest safety for blood pressure fluctuations. Use only a chair specifically designed for dialysis. Leave that beast of a recliner for another room—it's not the same thing!

2. What is the availability of necessary plumbing?

You will need a sink, bathtub, or toilet to secure the waste line hose—the plastic tube that will drain the used dialysis solution and waste produced by dialysis. You can connect two waste lines together, so the receptacle can be a fair distance away. Take care when you run a waste line that it won't kink or trip someone along its path. For tips for on how to create a simple pass-through in a wall to thread a waste line directly into a bathroom, see Appendix 3.

3. What does the patient want to do while dialyzing?

Do you want to be in the hub of your family's activity, like in a family room or TV room? Or would you rather be tucked away in the privacy of a study or guest bedroom? Choose your location based on your personal style and preference. Remember: doing dialysis at home gives you this type of flexibility and the capacity to take control of your situation as much as possible. Why not consider your own personal preferences? Steve, for example, has one non-negotiable requirement: a television.

#4. Does the dialysis helper have a comfortable place to work?

Dr. Thakur told us that doing Home Hemodialysis was sort of like boiling potatoes on the stove. You can do other things, but you must be close enough in case your potatoes boil over!

Linda works on her laptop computer during Steve's treatments; often, she pays bills or does other household chores—all within range to hear and respond to alarms. For overnight, extended dialysis treatments, Linda and Steve sleep in their own bed—with the dialysis machine humming alongside them.

5. Can emergency personnel easily reach the patient?

If your dialysis patient is particularly fragile with a heart condition or other medical condition that may require a call to the paramedics, consider this in your planning. Steve and Linda now use an alcove in their living room, for example. Part of the appeal of this room—in addition to the large television—is that it is on the first floor, and would be more easily accessible should Linda need to call 911. Their bedroom is on the second floor: sixteen stairs straight up, with a concrete landing below—not ideal for a fast trip on a gurney.

#6. What is your storage situation like?

As we've mentioned before, Home Dialysis requires space for plenty of equipment and supplies. But, as always, there are many space solutions. Some people store all their equipment in their dialysis room. Others have a separate storage area—even a clean garage or outdoor storage shed—and bring in adequate supplies for one or two treatments at a time.

Storage is so critical to smooth Home Dialysis, we have devoted an entire chapter to it. Check out our storage ideas in Chapter 10 before you set up your dialysis area. We can almost guarantee you will find some new solutions to your storage issues!

#7. How will your Hemodialysis room "flow?"

As you envision your dialysis area, plan for enough room for the helper to move easily around the patient and equipment. The helper's ease and comfort are important in making the process go smoothly. We've included space templates in Appendix 2 to help you map out your traffic flow as you prepare your design.

#8. Have you planned for waste and proper clean-up?

Dialysis generates waste in the form of paper and plastic—as well as fluid waste. Planning ahead for this makes the whole process easier. Here are some tips:

- Break down cardboard boxes. Cut the seams and flatten them for recycling as you go; otherwise, you'll have a pile of hazardous, bulky obstacles in your way. Bill Peckham, one of our heroes, advertises free cardboard boxes on Craig's List—and people gladly pick them up to use as sturdy moving boxes.

- Remember that "sharps" (needles from syringes, blood sugar testing lancets, and fistula needles) require "sharps containers." These are the hard plastic containers—usually red—that you can buy at your local pharmacy. Steve and Linda found that when using fistula needles, the large sharps containers which are over a foot tall are the most convenient. Sharps containers are taken back to the pharmacy when full, and disposed of as medical waste—for a small fee.

• Plan for large waste receptacles to be placed easily within reach. Steve and Linda use a large wicker laundry hamper lined with black garbage or yard waste bags from the local warehouse store. It saves steps to keep a stash of extra bags folded at the bottom of the container so you can immediately reline the waste receptacle after each use.

• Certain items such as plastic wrappers for large IV bags, cardboard, and the paper packaging for syringes can be recycled. Plan to have the appropriate bins so you handle each item only once.

• Combine similar items in a large basket or trunk. Steve and Linda use a hinged rattan basket from an import store (check Pier One or CostPlus) to hold a roll of black plastic yard waste bags, a roll of paper towels, and a plastic dispenser for antiseptic wipes. This simplifies clean-up at the end of each run.

• A washable area rug can be easily placed at the foot of the dialysis machine to give your own flooring some protection from blood or iodine spills. Roll or fold it up between uses and store in a basket or on your dialysis cart.

#9: Create a "station" for your pre- and post-dialysis monitoring.

You will require certain data from your patient before and after each Hemodialysis treatment. Keep needed items grouped together for your convenience.

You'll need:

- **Kilogram scale for pre- and post-dialysis weights. You may take the weight in pounds, but have a calculator nearby to convert pounds to kilograms (pounds divided by 2.2 = weight in kilograms). Of course, you will confirm your math with your instructor or doctor.**

- **Blood pressure cuff**

- **Blood sugar test kit, if applicable**

- **Clipboard with pen for recording your patient's data**

- **Extra batteries for automatic blood pressure cuff and scale**

- **Extra pens and log forms for recording your data.**

#10: Have you provided for safety and backup?

Don't start a Hemodialysis treatment without thinking: safety first! For each and every treatment, have the following equipment immediately at hand:

- **Always have a fully charged phone available—in case you need to reach a hotline or call 911. You may never need to call, but if you do, we promise you won't want to be hunting for the phone! Seconds can count.**

- **Have a rechargeable flashlight ready to go before starting any treatment that may take you beyond daylight hours. Steve and Linda keep a flashlight** charging in an electrical outlet right next to the dialysis machine, so it's always ready.

- If you live in an area of frequent power outages, you may want to consider a backup power generator. Ask your Home Dialysis educator about this.

- Have your instruction manual at the ready in case you come across an alarm signal you aren't familiar with.

- Keep your sheet of special instructions—how to perform an emergency rinseback or manual rinseback—in a consistent place, preferably on the shelf directly under the machine.

- Keep your "Clamp and Cut Kit" on the shelf under the machine as well. The Clamp and Cut Kit is the transparent pack with the supplies needed to get the dialysis patient off the machine and away from the house in a dire physical emergency such as an earthquake or a home fire. May you never, ever have to use that one!

- If you require specific supplies for your particular situation, keep them in a consistent place— immediately at hand. Steve has what he calls his "Heart Attack Kit:" a five-inch canvas bag containing his Nitroglycerine tablets and aspirin in case he has chest pain. But it's right there, in a consistent place, should he need the medication.

These, then, are the very basics for setting up your own "Hemodialysis Center!" Notice how much we talk about consistent, just-in-case preparations. Hopefully, you will never encounter anything so serious that you need the Clamp and Cut Kit, but it is smart and safe to think of these things in advance, and build them into your systems from the very beginning.

Now, let's turn to setting up your home for Peritoneal Dialysis. You will find similarities, though Peritoneal Dialysis is easier. First of all, you will not require a special chair or recliner.

For **Continuous Ambulatory Peritoneal Dialysis**, you will need the following:

- IV pole
- Dialysis solution bags and tubing
- Heating pad for warming your solution
- Cleansing materials as directed by your Center.

For **Continuous Cycling Peritoneal Dialysis**, you will need:

- Your cycler (machine) set on a bedside stand (Note: the cycler warms the dialysis solution through the night.)
- Dialysis solution and appropriate tubing
- Waste line running to an appropriate receptacle such as a sink or toilet, just as with Hemodialysis
- For both types of Peritoneal Dialysis, you will need:
- Storage for solution, tubing, and other supplies
- A system for keeping track of your weight and vital signs
- A system for ordering new supplies
- Garbage and recycling containers close at hand to make the process as effortless as it can be.

Is this all possible? Of course it is! It just takes some planning ahead and flexibility. Remember, the end result is an easier life for you and your family.

Part Two:
Bring In the Designer!

Chapter Six:

How a Designer Thinks

The whole point of design is to create a space that functions well for your specific needs. Design is also about style and appearance—and that's where people sometimes feel put off. On the surface, the concept of design may seem "snooty"—a frill that we regular folks don't have the luxury to think about. But when you consider that *the point of design is good function*—and that the way a space looks and feels can improve the quality of your life—design becomes an essential.

Designers are different. They think differently. They look at a physical space and see possibilities the rest of us wouldn't imagine. Many people believe that designers are unaffordable—and they certainly can be. But if you are working with the right designer—one who knows your resources and your specific goals—a designer can be very affordable, and actually save you money in costly mistakes. A good designer will look at what you have, and start from there. Linda was surprised at how often Jane tapped resources like the Goodwill, Value Village, Target, Marshalls, Ross, and Costco. Don't make the common mistake of being intimidated by the whole idea before you start. Besides, we've brought *you* a designer for the cost of this book!

A good designer knows there are many ways to economize on any project. Knowing what to spend money on—and where to economize—is a big part of the job.

Let's take color, for example. Painting is one of the least expensive modifications you can make to create visual change and enhance the mood of a room. A gallon of paint can give you a lot of pizzazz for a relatively small amount of money. Remember that one can of paint usually costs the same as another. You can buy a soothing, relaxing color—or one that jangles your nerves—for exactly the same price! The difference is in the design. You can also achieve the effect of a color (how it makes you feel) by painting only one or two walls rather than the whole room. As a general rule, kicking off your room make-over with a fresh coat of paint is a good place to start—and it's cost-effective. We'll go into color and how it makes you feel in another chapter.

Another great way to save money is to "shop at home" first. Furniture and finishing touches can come from what you already have. A light sanding and a couple of coats of spray paint can freshen and revitalize a functional piece of furniture that you may have banished to your garage or basement.

However, if you truly need new things, check out the IKEA catalog. Their slogan, "You don't have to be rich, just smart!" applies particularly when it comes to their cabinets and shelving units. Jane found IKEA's shelving prices, quality, and scale perfect for the Home Dialysis space. In fact, the room diagrams in this book were developed using IKEA shelving as the model.

Don't forget about places like furniture consignment stores and import stores like Pier One or CostPlus. Check out any furniture store with the word "outlet" in the title. And never write off Target,

Marshall's, Ross, TJ Maxx, and warehouse stores like Costco and Sam's Club for small home furnishings and textiles.

Remember that it is the designer's intention to create a room and home that will work effectively for you and the specific requirements of your life. If you aren't happy with the results, it isn't a successful design! When the work is done well, the end result should truly feel like "coming home."

Chapter Seven:

A Designer Figures Out—*With You*— What You Want and Need to Do

Just like a good doctor meeting you for the first time, a good designer gets to know something about you and what you need. Some of your needs in designing your Home Dialysis space will be fairly obvious: you need to create a functional space where dialysis can be performed with as much comfort, safety, and efficiency as possible.

A designer would also want to know who lives in the home: is this a home of a boomer couple or a home with young children? What is the flavor of your lifestyle: quietly traditional, casual contemporary, soccer-mom chic? Do you have plenty of room to work with, or are you already feeling the pinch of limited space? Are you a neat and organized person, or are you drowning in clutter?

We outlined in Chapter 5 the very basics for putting together a workable Home Dialysis room. You may want to refer back to this information from time to time as we continue.

Here are the assumptions: you want to create a space that feels comfortable—not only for the person on dialysis, but for the rest of the family. Safe, smooth dialysis runs are a priority for you. You require careful attention to Storage Solutions (refer to Chapter 10).

You share the goal of minimizing the impact of dialysis on your life overall. Stated differently, we assume that you want dialysis to be a part of your life—but not consume it entirely.

Deciding Where to Dialyze

First of all, you will want to establish where you will dialyze. If you are doing overnight runs, that question is generally answered easily: in the bedroom. If, however, you are not doing overnight dialysis, we encourage you to find a room other than your bedroom. As we explain later, we encourage you to protect that bedroom as your private hideout, tucked away from the rest of the world.

If you are not dialyzing in bed, you will need to use a specially designed dialysis chair. This is a recliner-style chair that enables you to tip the patient way back in the event of low blood pressure. Do not use the family recliner; it's not the same. Standard dimensions of a dialysis chair are 32" wide by 47" deep by 48" high. But remember to allow for the full extension of the chair (74"), which then expands the space required to an area of about 32" wide by 74" deep by 48" high. Plan for a full extension of seven feet. You will also need to allow for room to work on either side of the dialysis chair, so all in all, plan for a

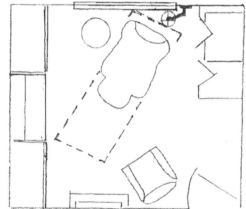

Dialysis chair full extension "footprint" as it relates to the room size and furnishings.

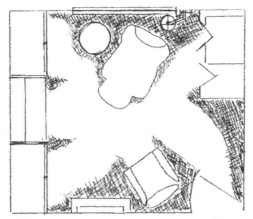

Highlighted areas indicating caregiver walk space as it relates to room, furnishings and storage access.

total dimension of 7.5 feet by 9 feet for the footprint of the dialysis chair and the helper's workspace.

In setting up a dialysis chair, allow space for another comfortable chair for the helper. Consider all the possibilities below:

Family Room:

This is the perfect spot for the patient who wants to be in the middle of family activities. Using a family room, however, may depend on the comfort level of the rest of the family. Admittedly, the sight of the medical paraphernalia can be jarring at first—but it becomes the new normal in short order.

Guest Room:

While a guest room is typically small to moderate in size, it could certainly accommodate a dialysis chair, a comfortable chair for the helper, and plenty of storage. You might want to consider using a day bed or futon instead of a full or queen bed for your guests. Linda once used a Murphy bed to optimize the function of a guest room. While expensive (several thousand dollars), today's Murphy beds are comfortable—and

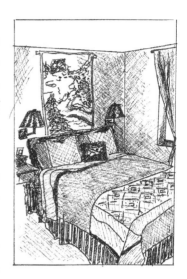

they can be built with custom cabinetry which would be ideal for a dialysis room. Linda's was financed through a home equity loan and enhanced the value of her home on resale.

Above: Guest bedroom 'before' being converted for use as a dialysis room. Below: Guest bedroom 'after' conversion to a dialysis room with examples of floor plan, wall elevations, and perspectives of the room conversion.

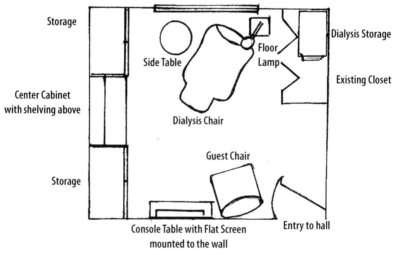

Room Size: 9 foot 7½ inches wide by 11 foot 3 inches long (drawings not to scale)

South wall elevation

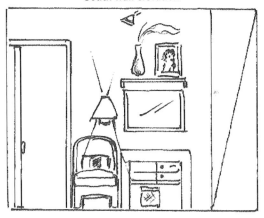

South Wall Perspective

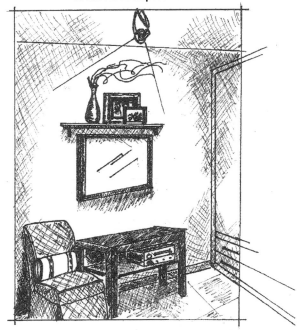

West Wall

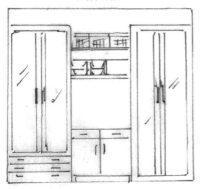

North Wall

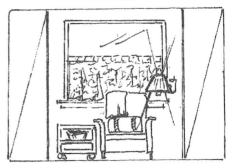

The diagonal lines on each side of this illustration indicate looking at the side (end) view of a wall or cabinet.

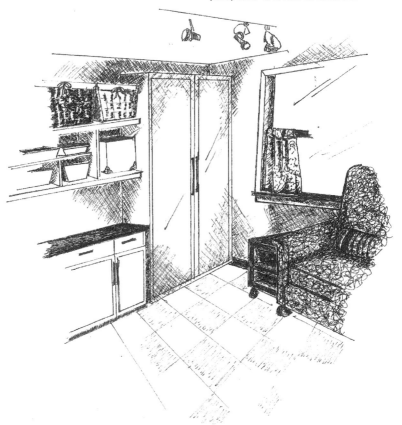

Dining Room:

You probably wouldn't think of using a dining room as a dialysis space but if your dining room is used mainly for special occasions—and you use a kitchen or other space for your regular family meals, a dining room could be a very practical space solution. It's interesting that the traditional dining room tends to be one of the least utilized rooms in homes today. Jane has devised some great methods for concealing the dialysis machine when not in use, so give the dining room some thought.

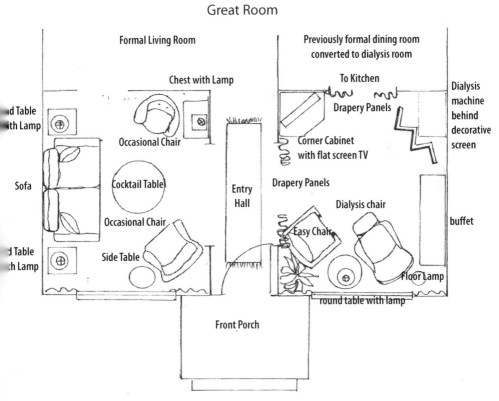

Room Size: 10 foot by 12 foot long (drawings not to scale)

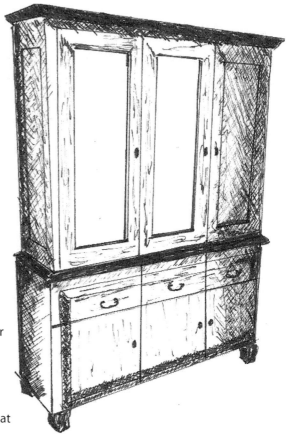

A dining room hutch and buffet can be repurposed as an interim storage solution. Using a static cling vinyl on the hutch glass to create a frosted look, or by lining the glass panels with an attractive fabric, the upper shelves can be used for medical supplies. The lower buffet cabinet is a perfect spot for dialysate solution storage. Keep in mind all this is a temporary repurposing and can be put back to it's original condition when that kidney transplant occurs!

Den or Home Office:

Like a guest room, this may be a very convenient space, especially if you plan to work while dialyzing. A den may have plenty of room for a dialysis chair, helper's chair, and good storage possibilities, too.

Bedroom:

Check out Jane's floor plan for a bedroom dialysis area, with privacy screening.

Remember to keep an open mind as you consider where to dialyze. There may be more than one space that could work for you. You may also want to re-think who occupies each room as dialysis moves home. A room switch may work better for everyone concerned. Be creative in re-thinking your home's spaces.

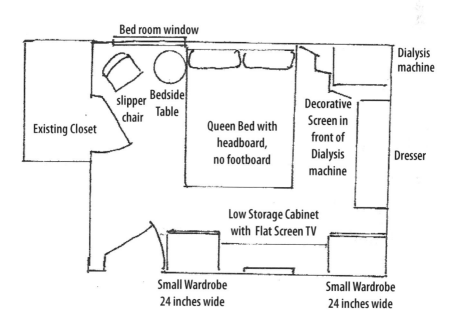

Room Size: 11 foot long by 8.5 foot wide (drawings not to scale)

Taking Measurements

After deciding where you want to dialyze, the next step is to take a careful set of measurements of your room dimensions. This can be a little tedious. But omitting this step can lead to a multitude of costly mistakes.

So, enlist the help of a friend or your partner and grab a metal, retractable tape measure—the kind you'd buy at Home Depot. Record all measurements, and take them with you when you go shopping.

Use the blank templates we have included in this book (Appendix 2) to map your existing space. Be sure to record doorways and the direction the door swings. Don't forget to record jogs or irregularities in the footprint of the room. Jane recommends that you record every dimension in both feet and inches, to save you time when ordering furniture, storage items, and draperies.

When you've done this step, measure all windows—including the height of the sill from the floor, and the inner and outer dimensions of every window. Make a note of the location of the electrical outlets and phone jacks.

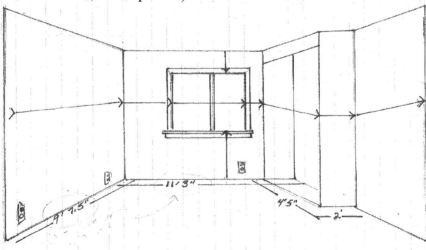

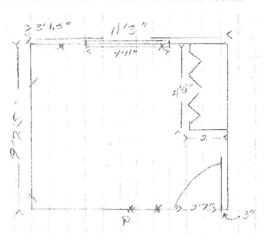

Measure and record the footprint dimensions for any furniture pieces you plan on using in the dialysis space.

How to Measure a Room

1st - Draw the four lines that comprise overall length and width of the room on graph paper (Appendix 2).

2nd - Now add all the areas where the walls change, i.e. closet walls, recesses in the walls, door entry to the room and windows.

3rd - Place small x's on the floor-plan drawing to remind yourself where the electrical outlets, cable and phone jacks are located.

To begin taking room measurements, start in one corner of the room. Continue in one direction around all four walls. Measure to inside edges of door and window opening to accurately place them on your drawing. (See example drawing.) Measure and insert nooks, recesses or other changes to the room walls.

Clearing Out What You Don't Need

Almost every redo begins with a good clean-out. Clean and clear out your room or space so you can use it well for its new purpose. Experts advise you to start this process armed and ready with three boxes for sorting:

- Things to keep
- Things to throw away or recycle
- Things to sell or give away

It will become obvious to you that you will need every square inch of storage space you can get, so be brutally honest about what you do and don't need.

Now, it's time to begin the design process! Let's move on to the creative—and more fun—parts!

Chapter Eight:

Designing the Furniture Layout

In Appendix 2, you will find a set of graph paper grids to map out your room's footprint with dimensions measured in feet and inches. We have also included traceable furniture templates with standard measurements for basic pieces of furniture—including your dialysis chair and dialysis machine.

We remind you that when you are using templates—even though they are based on standard measurements—be sure to check your furniture and space measurements. Don't make assumptions here, or you could be disappointed.

Templates do make the design process easier, particularly when you are weighing several options for your space.

Start with the Basics

You know that your space will require the following key pieces:

- **Dialysis chair**
- **Dialysis machine on its cart**

- Comfortable chair for helper
- Station for monitoring pre- and post-dialysis weights and blood pressures.

Using your floor plan template, draw the outline of your room. Then, use your furniture templates to lay out your dialysis room as described below.

Establish a Focal Point

The first thing to establish—after you draw your room's dimensions—is the room's *focal point.* This may be a fireplace, a view window, an entertainment center or (most typically) the wall that houses a flat-screen TV.

Arrange your key piece first

Your key piece is your largest piece. For this purpose, the key piece will likely be your dialysis chair. Arrange the key piece so that it faces your focal point. The key piece doesn't have to face the focal point squarely. Based on your room's floor space and the necessary room required to access the dialysis chair from both sides (approximately 30" on each side, expanding to 36" if allowing for wheel chair accessibility), it could mean that the dialysis chair is placed on a diagonal in relation to the focal point.

We want to emphasize the point of planning for the dialysis chair to be fully extended or reclined—configured as it is when it occupies the most space. This is a matter of safety. If you need to tip your patient back to stabilize blood pressure, you must be able to recline the chair fully—without hitting another piece of furniture or a wall!

Again, plan for an estimated 7.5 feet by 9 feet for your dialysis chair and maneuverability footprint.

Add your other pieces

After placing your "key piece," use cut-out furniture templates to add the other pieces you will need. We encourage you to add them to your floor plan even if you don't presently own the exact item you need. This might include another chair, an entertainment center, end table, floor lamp or desk and chair. Visualizing and making a list of these pieces will help in your planning. It also serves as a guide for helping others who want to help you, or maybe find pieces for you.

Once you've found a furniture configuration that you like, scan or copy your work. Then, remove your cut-outs—and start again! Try another configuration, thinking out of the box. Try anything—there's no harm in experimenting on paper.

Decide where the waste line will go

The waste line must feed into a sink, bathtub, or toilet to drain. When choosing a dialysis location, consider the following:

- **Is there a sink, toilet, or tub in the room, or in an adjoining room. See Jane's tip for cutting through a wall to make an easy waste line tunnel. Don't attempt this yourself, however, unless you have the appropriate skill set. (See Appendix 3.)**

- **Is there a wet bar in a recreation room or family room?**

- **Is there an adjoining laundry area? Again, think of Jane's trick of tunneling through the wall.**

Remember that two waste lines can be connected together to create an even longer line.

Add Storage!

Because it's such a confounding issue with Home Dialysis, we have devoted an entire chapter to storage. Please refer to Chapter 10 for a complete discussion of these ideas, and then return and add your storage areas into your template floor plans.

There *will* be Waste!

Plan for convenient placement of trash receptacles. Steve and Linda use generous wicker hampers with lids, lined with plastic garbage bags for safe disposal. You may wish to have another similar receptacle for recyclable materials, such as cardboard, paper and plastic. You will also need appropriate "sharps" containers for discarding needles.

We will deal with color, lighting, accessories, and finishing touches just a bit later. But start with the basic needs, and then move on from there.

Chapter Nine:

Taking Inventory of What You Have; Adding What You Need

Taking a furniture and furnishings inventory is the next important step and isn't as boring as it sounds. One expert suggested thinking about this as if you are taking a shopping trip in your own home. After all, the price is right! Include your entire home in your "shopping trip." Inventory all rooms, not just the room you are planning to use for dialysis. Include all dressers, office credenzas, buffets, bookcases, and shelving units.

Browse through all garage areas and storage facilities. Items you once banished may be repurposed, given your new circumstances. A perfect example of furniture reincarnation is the classic entertainment center: the kind designed to house a large tube TV—now nearly obsolete. These entertainment centers can be perfectly redirected for use in dialysis and dialysis-related storage. Many older pieces require only a simple cleaning. Others will require a light sanding and a few coats of spray paint; solid black or white can be very versatile.

Record the measurements of all likely candidates.

Now, can you identify something special—maybe a framed picture, a photo, an area rug, a vase, a throw, a décor pillow, a decorative box—that your patient particularly likes? Something that always makes them feel comfortable to look at or touch? Something that reminds them of a great vacation or other special event? Anything that resonates or touches your heart. This type of object is important for two reasons.

First, it is critical to surround yourself with things you enjoy—especially when your life feels so complicated. Your favorite object becomes sort of a touchstone to remind you that you're still hanging in there.

Second, a favorite object can be the foundation of your color choice, and it serves as the design reference and your inspiration or jumping off point.

To review:

- **Shop your own home first**

- **Make a note of objects that are special to you**

- **Make a note of the colors that attract your eye**

- **List all objects available for you to use.**

When it's time to go shopping—outside your home—make a list of:

- **Essentials: things you absolutely need to set up the Home Dialysis space**

- **Items that will help make the environment more comfortable or attractive.**

- Be sure your shopping list includes: rechargeable flashlight, roll of duct tape, antiseptic wipes and garbage bags.

Where does a designer shop?

Jane says that for larger items, she starts with furniture consignment stores. These typically contain cast-offs of superior quality—things that people spent too much money on to just give away. You can find tremendous bargains in such shops. Check your yellow pages or the Internet under "furniture consignment" dealers.

Besides consignment shops, here's where the real bargains are:

- Garage sales
- Salvage shops, particularly for cabinetry
- Any furniture store with the word "outlet" in its name
- Thriftshops: Goodwill Industries, Value Village, Salvation Army
- For new items, particularly when good storage is required, Jane shops IKEA. Their take-along catalogs will allow you to plan efficiently. In addition, the IKEA pieces are nice enough that you will still use them in your home when dialysis is no longer required, like after that new kidney comes!

For finishing touches, Jane recommends the following:

- Shop your own home first
- TJ Maxx, Marshall's, Ross

- **Garage sales**
- **Import shops like CostPlus or Pier One**
- **Warehouse stores like Costco or Sam's Club.**

The point is to find bargains that work to make your life easier and more comfortable, and your space more attractive. Let's go on to Chapter 10, and the issue of storage.

Chapter Ten:

Storage Solutions

Storage is a big deal in the world of Home Dialysis. While a dialysis chair and machine take up some space, you'll quickly find that it's the rest of the supplies—particularly the bags of solution—that require special planning.

Plan your space so that supplies are close at hand. Ideally, you will have supplies for three to five runs in the room, with the remainder of your monthly supplies within a reasonable distance.

Let's start with the dialysate bags

Dialysis solution (dialysate) for Hemodialysis comes shipped in two five-liter bags per cardboard box. Peritoneal Dialysis bags will vary in size according to the patient's dialysis prescription, but they also come packed in cardboard boxes. You can stack the boxes if you have the room, but removing some of them from the cardboard boxes will save you time. A step saved is a step toward sanity!

It isn't recommended that you stack the bags, but you can nestle them together side-by-side for the most efficient use of space. You will need shelves made of smooth surfaces. We like melamine—it's smooth and easily cleaned. Don't use wire shelving for bags. For

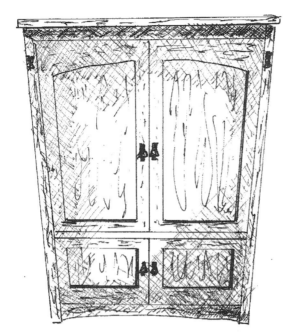

A large entertainment armoire like this one has become nearly obsolete with the arrival of the flat screen TV. But it can be a perfect storage unit for dialysate bags, just by adding extra shelves.

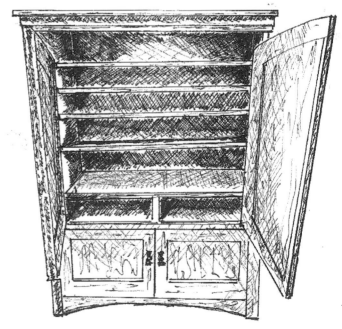

Home Hemodialysis, shelves need to be a minimum of 15" deep, but 18" works even better. Out of their cardboard boxes, the dialysate bags measure 13" wide and are about 8.25" thick.

Cartridges, Tubing, and Saline—Oh My!

You will receive approximately one month's worth of supplies from your local kidney center. Careful storage will allow for a reliable inventory. Shelving units, dressers, and armoires are great ideas for storing these items.

See an excellent example of a Storage Wall Unit Jane has designed, with all specifications included, in Appendix 4. If not perfect for your needs, it will at least be adaptable, and give you some good ideas. Plus, it can be easily repurposed later if you move or your patient gets a kidney transplant.

Keep Shelving Units Safe

Shelving units can help with a variety of functions, but remember these specific safety tips:

- **Load heavy items onto the lower shelves and lighter items (like Chux underpads) overhead**

- **Anchor shelving units to the wall to earthquake-proof your space**

- **Provide a step stool to discourage any shelf-climbers!**

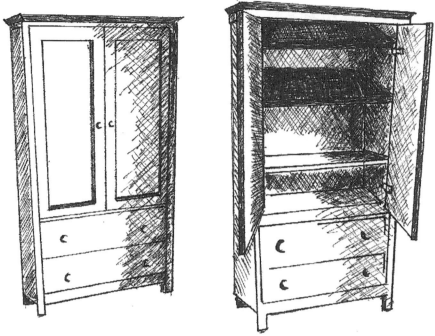

One patient suggested that an armoire could feature shelves which are slightly tipped downward. Theoretically, one could connect dialysate bags directly from the shelving unit without hanging them onto an IV pole. If you try this, be sure that your dialysis machine is close enough to the storage unit so it doesn't put extra stretch on the tubing—and that your bags empty completely during treatment.

Create Individual Supply Packets

Linda swears by Daily Packs: gallon sized zip-lock style bags which contain all of the small items required for a day's dialysis run. Each pack includes the required number of syringes, four-by-four gauze pads, catheter caps, alcohol and iodine wipes, and the like.

She also uses Weekly Packs: items re-used through the week like a multi-use vial of Heparin, paper and plastic tape. The work saved in running to gather supplies for each run is substantial.

Use Baskets for Storage and Décor

Baskets are useful, attractive and come in a wide variety of sizes, shapes, and prices. Jane hung a beautiful rattan tote bag on Steve's wall to hold an entire month's supply of dialysis fistula needles. Think of generous wicker laundry hampers and large lidded baskets with ample storage space. Similarly, sturdy canvas boxes or file boxes can be functional and attractive.

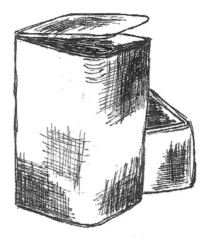

Tall baskets with hinged lids can be used for much more than clothing hampers. They make a perfect option for storing Chux or other bulky items. A matching basket used elsewhere in the room lends a sense of continuity and repetition of texture.

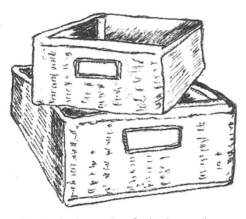

Nesting baskets or low flat baskets make good options for organizing remote controls and other table top clutter.

Chapter Eleven:

Using Color to Make the
Dialysis Room More Comfortable

Color is a powerful tool in the world of design. We all know instinctively that some colors make us feel tense and irritable, while other colors comfort and soothe us. Have you ever walked into a beautiful room and felt your blood pressure ease, your pulse rate slow down, and your mind go "Ahhh!"—in an unconscious sigh of relief? What a wonderful feeling!

If you have any question about this, explore the Internet for luxury hotels and spas. Look at the colors they choose to promote that feeling of warmth, that calm sense that everything is going to be okay. You'll notice that such spas use soft, neutral colors overall—and use bolder accent colors for interest.

Color can be complicated to work with, and it's easy to make a mistake. You may know this firsthand if you've ever labored over paint color swatches and discovered that the two-inch sample you loved in the store looked awful on your wall!

Designers like Jane spend hours taking classes in color theory. They study lighting and the way colors interact with light. Jane says the human eye can actually discern ninety-three million variations of color! Thankfully, there are only twenty thousand color variations available among paint retailers.

A trained designer can detect shades and subtleties of color the rest of us might not notice. We may not know how to make the best color selections, but we are able to recognize a finished product we like.

Let's talk for a moment about color and its relation to light. The natural lighting available in the room is the single most important thing to consider when selecting a paint color. The paint color you choose will interact with natural lighting by day—and with incandescent lighting by night. How your chosen color "plays" with light will determine how happy you are with your paint job.

A southern-facing room with lots of large windows provides abundant natural light for the biggest part of the day. These rooms will naturally look and feel warmer. It follows that northern-facing rooms that never get direct natural sunlight feel cooler. West-facing rooms provide intense sunlight for the late afternoon, and consequently heat up the room toward the end of the day. East-facing windows are bathed in natural light in the morning.

Surprisingly, Jane tells us that colors cut with gray (technically called burnt sienna and/or raw umber) have a better chance of turning out to look the way you'd envisioned them in your room. (In Designer-Speak, they "read" better.) This is especially true if you are drawn to bright or vivid colors. If your room has a lot of natural light, bright colors become even more vivid, whereas a more gray or "cut" version of that color has a better chance of reading to your eye as the color you originally envisioned. (This whole concept of gray-cut colors skated high over Linda's head, but she certainly agreed Jane was correct when she viewed the finished product.)

Because we often just know what we like—but haven't a clue how to create it, we have elected not to get too deep into color theory. To spare us—and to save us precious time—Jane has included samples of several different palettes using colors from Benjamin Moore Paints. She chose this company because Benjamin Moore offers a quality product: easy to apply, with a wonderful range of shade options, and a number of washable finishes to choose from. If you would like get larger color swatches—always a good idea, you can order them at your local paint store using the identifying number on each swatch (Refer also to Appendix 6).

On page 130 you will find a table of Jane's favorite color combinations and examples of colors that have worked beautifully in a variety of interiors.

Use the lighter color in each color family for walls. Select the darker colors—"hues" in Designer-Speak—for your accent colors. Feel free to mix and match among the color families; they'll look great. Remember that it's easier to change accent pieces than the main color.

Are there other colors that could work well? Certainly—but the themes Jane has chosen are universal and dependable. You won't likely go wrong with any of these. If the idea of painting seems impossible to you, remember that painting even only one or two walls can make a difference. Plus, painting is a job that can be delegated to that great handy-person who is begging for a way to help you.

What if your favorite color is a bright red or blue, and you really want to use it in your new dialysis room? Remember that bright, strong saturated colors may actually make your room feel more energized, but it can backfire on you. Your room may feel overwhelmed by color—not at all what you want when your dialysis patient is already feeling confined to the machine.

A better option for using those stronger colors would be as accents: décor pillows, an area rug, a comfy throw, lamp base, accessory, drapery panels, or art pieces. It's all about achieving balance in the mix of color and items you choose for your room.

When you think about color combinations or palettes, ask yourself the following:

- **Is there one palette which says "Pick me"?**
- **Do you have an emotional response—positive or negative—to any?**
- **Is there one you already know would get boring or old quickly?**
- **Is there a palette that you simply don't like?**

We think you will find Jane's sample color palettes inviting and easy to work with. In each color family, notice the two lighter colors will work best for walls. Again, the darker hues can be used as accents like pillows, curtains, pictures, throw rugs. Don't be afraid to mix and match from among the sample color families.

For the next few days or weeks, pay attention to your reaction to color. If, for example, you are able to visit a spa or other relaxing environment, notice the colors that are used. Likewise, if you are in an environment that makes your skin crawl—or generally makes you tense—pay attention to those colors, too. Clip out magazine photos of scenes or rooms you instinctively like. A designer can help you take these observations and translate them into a color palette that will work for you.

We've suggested in an earlier chapter the concept of selecting a specific item of particular comfort to your patient: a favorite picture, décor pillow, throw, area rug. The idea was partly to use this object as a jumping off point in beginning your color selections. Use the objects you love to guide your color selection, and you will likely find your entire environment to be more pleasing. Keep in mind that each decision for your room counts: from wall color to fabrics, from wood tones to the cover on your dialysis chair—if it doesn't harmonize with your jumping off point, go with something that does.

Chapter Twelve:

Privacy: Disguising the Elephant

Do you remember the childhood song that went "One of these things is not like the other..."? It was designed to help children pick out the one object in a group that stood out like a sore thumb.

In your home, a dialysis machine will probably never look like it fits in. Of course it cannot be disguised during a treatment. But depending on which room you're using for dialysis, you may want to camouflage the machine when it's not in use.

Here are Jane's never-fail ideas for disguising that "elephant" in your home!

Screens

Movable multi-panel screens can be very versatile. Look for rattan screens in import stores. Jane found a white wicker screen that didn't work with the existing décor in Steve and Linda's bedroom, but the size was perfect and price was right. She then used a solid neutral color bed sheet (really) to cover the back of the screen so the wicker wouldn't show through when it was sitting in front of the window above the dialysis machine. She then covered the front of the screen with a smart-looking IKEA fabric that picked up the colors in the décor pillows on the bed. Jane "upholstered"—fastened—the whole thing together with a staple gun. The outcome was a perfect accessory that completely disguised the dialysis machine and added an attractive new layer of visual interest to the master bedroom.

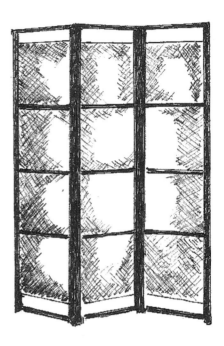

Screens come in many finishes, styles, and price points. Shoji screens, for example, are very versatile, and work with any number of room styles. Asian design pieces mix with almost anything.

Don't overlook the Internet when shopping for a decorative screen. Type in "interior decorative screens" and you'll find a whole raft of options.

Drapery Panels

Ready-made drapery panels are not just for the windows! Drapery panels can be the handiest and least expensive way to mask a large area concealing the clutter of medical supplies (or anything else, for that matter), divide up a room without major construction, or add another option for privacy.

Drapery panels come in a variety of colors, styles, and fabrics. They are one of the easiest ways to add texture and color to a room.

A standard panel size is 45" wide by 86" long. Oversized drapery panels are harder to find; IKEA has some panels that are 45" wide by 110" long and can be hemmed to your desired length. Of course, anything can by custom-ordered, but that costs a lot more.

In Steve and Linda's home, Jane hung a tension rod and a rich black "rod-pocket" drapery panel from Bed, Bath, & Beyond over an alcove in a tiny office space just outside the bedroom. They were able to stack over thirty dialysis solution boxes all the way to the ceiling! But the black panel made the alcove seem to disappear from view.

In another location, where there was a storage space with an opening too wide for standard hardware, Jane suspended a rod from the ceiling on slender wires. Using extra-long, lightweight drapery panels, the effect was that of a floor-to-ceiling window.

The same trick was applied to a large walk-in closet space that had no doors. The space—even on the rare occasions that it was somewhat organized—was a clutter magnet. But the lovely light-weight faux silk panels added a rich disguise and transformed an eyesore into a pleasing segue from the bathroom into the bedroom.

One of the best budget buys in Jane's arsenal of drapery options are bed sheets! You can't beat their price for pure yardage. So when she's in a pinch, you'll find Jane shopping the clearance items in the bedding department. Twin-sized flat bed sheets make excellent drapery panels. Hang them from drapery rings equipped with little clips that snap directly onto the fabric, and you're good to go!

Drapery Installations as Room Dividers

Have you ever noticed the curtains on tracks that hospitals use to partition off segments of a room to provide privacy? We've all seen these in patient rooms or emergency rooms; sometimes, they're used in operating room waiting areas.

The tracks are a product called KS Systems. They're light and practical, and they maximize the utility of the space available.

The cost of this option is relatively inexpensive (about $3 per running foot). The system can hang long expanses of draperies, and the tracks can be curved for custom-fit solutions. Mounted on the ceiling, this system can provide the perfect answer for draping off large sections of a room.

Jane has used KS Systems in a great room where she had to find a budget solution for an area that required over twenty-two feet of floor-to-ceiling draperies. To complicate things further, there were curves: two convex and one concave. But light-weight and flexible, KS Systems worked.

KS Systems are not available through general retailers, but can be purchased through an interior designer. IKEA has recently released a similar product.

While this may sound like an institutional-looking solution, fabric selection makes all the difference.

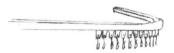

KS Systems for hanging window treatments as well as being utilized for hanging fabrics as room dividers. While KS Systems are available through interior designers, IKEA has a very similar product available.

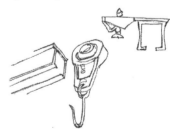

Chapter Thirteen:

Lighting Tricks Designers Use

Lighting is critical in creating an efficient, functional, and aesthetically pleasing space. Poor lighting design can make a space feel unwelcoming. It's unflattering to your appearance and can be stress-inducing. But good lighting design produces a sense of comfort and accessibility. Steve and Linda noticed this nearly every time they'd walk into a treatment center, emergency room, or ICU room. Glaring, overhead lights—usually in that nerve-jangling fluorescent variety—seem to spoil nearly every such environment. That may add to the stress we feel in medical environments.

From a designer's perspective, Jane compartmentalizes lighting as follows:

Midrange lighting

This is the ambient lighting provided by table lamps, usually at about eighteen inches above the surface of an end table. Floor lamps can provide the same function. These lamps provide light and visual warmth at the middle range of your room. But notice that these aren't the glaring, in-your-face fluorescent variety.

Task lighting

Task lights come in all shapes, sizes, and price ranges. IKEA has excellent, affordable examples. Task lighting provides the high-intensity, all-business lighting you need when you are starting a Home Dialysis treatment, drawing up important medications such as Heparin, and—above all—when you are troubleshooting a problem. Steve and Linda have a floor lamp with three separate "spotlights." The beauty of this lamp is that they can use only one light—or all three, and the lights can be manually directed to the task at hand.

Task lighting for use during dialysis and curling up with a good book.

Accent lighting for art pieces

Designers often use accent lighting to highlight framed art. If you have a piece of art that means a great deal to you, adding an art light is a small and dynamic way to emphasize the piece.

Art lights can be accessed at IKEA for as little as $15 or so, and through other lighting retailers for more than $50. The difference they make to your wall art adds a lovely addition to your room.

Uplighting

Jane places small canister lights—priced at only five or six dollars apiece—on the floor to beautify a plant, a silk ficus tree, or art object. You don't see the little lamp. Instead, you do see the effect that packs a big visual punch for very little money.

Natural lighting

Allowing as much natural light into a room as possible is always a mood booster. If the view out the window isn't wonderful, consider using translucent, light-diffusing sheer curtains. They give a soft filtered glow to a room while masking any exterior visual distractions.

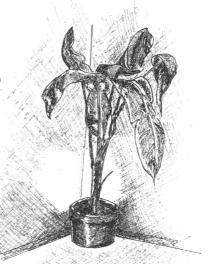

Uplighting adds drama, visual interest and depth to a room.

Overhead lighting

Recessed ceiling can lighting provides the best and most even overhead light distribution. Recessed lighting is usually installed with a dimmer switch that provides light level flexibility.

A single fixture in the center of the ceiling is much more common in older construction. If this is what you have to work with, you will find mid-range table lamps and floor lamp lighting that much more important.

Reflected light

Providing reflected light is a technique for creating the feeling of additional light sources in a room. Adding mirrors can accomplish this. When placed on adjacent or opposite walls, mirrors give the effect of having an additional window to bring the natural beauty of the outdoors into your room.

Mirrored surfaces in a room serve to cast light in interesting ways at different times of the day and evening. A piece of mirrored furniture used as a side table, polished metals for accents and accessories, glass table tops, crystal tear drops on accessories or lamps are all sources of reflected light.

Linda's non-designer favorite—the flashlight

Linda couldn't resist the opportunity to remind people to always have a charged flashlight or shop light immediately available for each dialysis run.

Chapter Fourteen:

Finishing Touches:
Cost Conscious Designer Secrets

If you've gotten this far in your room design, sit down and put your feet up. What an accomplishment! It's important to remember that this is a process, and can be a lot of work. Going through these steps, however, will ensure a more relaxed, balanced, and emotionally satisfying experience with Home Dialysis.

It's time to ask the designer for the special touches that finish off the room, and make it feel comfortable, polished, and really pulled together.

Here are Jane's favorite ideas:

- **Use accessories to your best advantage**
- **Try to use fewer—but larger—accessories.**
- **Group larger accessories and smaller ones together to create arrangements.**

Use the "rule of odd numbers" when creating table top accessories or wall collages. Groupings of three, five, seven, etc. are somehow more pleasing to the eye.

Long, curly willow branches bundled together make expensive-looking wall accessories, but can also look great in a floor vase or bucket. Craft stores and import stores often carry these.

Bring in your color accents

Assuming you have found an overall soothing color for your room, it's time to accent with décor pillows, comfy throws, photographs, art, candles, or favorite objects from your travels. Remember: the last five percent of what's done to your room will add the biggest visual impact—so surround yourself with the colors and things you love.

Texturize your room

Texture adds richness to a room, making it look more polished—and more expensive. Fabrics give us a variety of ways to accomplish this. Think in terms of nubby woven throws in combination with inexpensive polyester silk décor pillows. Colorful canvas boxes or sturdy rattan baskets sitting on open shelving add an element of texture, while providing functional storage solutions. Window treatments, such as drapery panels layered over woven wood shades or sheers, add texture. Adding texture works most effectively when you use different textures in three or four different ways in the same room: layering the room with visual interest.

Metal touches add "bling" to a room

A mirror frame in a metallic finish, a lamp base in a polished chrome, a bronze vase, a grouping of silver picture frames or silver boxes add terrific "bling." Think of these little touches as jewelry for your space.

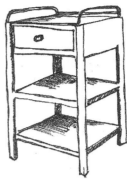

A small scale metal table with a drawer and two shelves makes a perfect end table option. Not only is it easy to clean should there be a spill, but it adds close-at-hand storage options.

Add plants

Bring the outdoors in. Green plants make an area feel more vibrant, but they don't have to be real. Silk plants are now so affordable—and beautiful—they can fool even the most discriminating eye. Uplight them using inexpensive canister lights.

Plants bring the outdoors in and add a wonderful 'life force' to any room. No need to overdo it, one or two will work just fine.

Bring in warmth

You've heard it all before, but we'll repeat it here once again. Soft furnishings: upholstered ottomans, chairs, décor pillows, throws, area rugs, wall hangings soften a room and make it feel warm and cozy. Placing an area rug on top of your existing carpet anchors a room. An area rug is the perfect place to begin when you formulate your color palette.

De-Clutter!

Planning ahead to keep your space uncluttered will keep your room looking comfortable and your dialysis runs more efficient. Find a nice basket, for example, for the phone, and those three necessary TV clickers. That way, you'll always know where to find them—but the area will look uncluttered, too. Small items like nail clippers, emery boards, tissues, and pens and paper can be grouped in a drawer or basket next to the dialysis chair—to keep them out of sight while still within reach.

Provide adequate waste receptacles

They can be pretty, like lined woven baskets, for instance. Laundry hampers, particularly baskets, are perfect in appearance and function.

An extra-large woven waste basket with a matching lid mixes right in with the room décor.

Group pictures or objects together.

When decorating a table top, mantle, or shelf, group things together. Be sure the objects are of different heights for the best effect. As we've said, many designers use odd numbers of objects for a more pleasing appearance. Use similarly colored frames for all your favorite photos. They'll look more like a purposeful collection and less like a jumble.

Add music!

Don't forget to add a radio or CD player—some source of music—to create a mood that's comfortable for you.

Part Three:
All-Around Tricks for Living Better With Home Dialysis

Chapter Fifteen:

The Home Hemodialysis "Comfort Kit"

The Home Hemodialysis patient must stay in one place—on the hose—for a period of two to four hours. There's no way to move, and certainly no way to get up and get something you might want or need. It's kind of like when the Captain keeps the seatbelt light on for the whole flight. (As a matter of fact, we've found some great ideas from companies targeting travelers!)

So, how can we make the dialysis time more comfortable for the patient?

First, we can provide a comfortable physical space—the focus of the design work we've discussed already. But on a more personal level, what does the dialysis patient need right at hand?

In the best of all worlds, each dialysis patient would have a Comfort Kit or basket within easy reach. And while all patients are different, we've assembled a list of things that might make the process easier for many. Wouldn't it be great if each Home Dialysis patient received a Comfort Kit as a gift?

In the Comfort Kit we recommend, we've considered components that address physical comfort—including thirst and the overall sensation of dryness which many dialysis patients experience. We've also considered intellectual stimulation because the two-to-four hour stretches can be boring. And, we've considered relaxation. Here are some suggestions for your Home Dialysis Comfort Kit (Refer to Appendix l):

Providing for Physical Comfort

Again, take a tip from the travel industry. When you think of it, products for airline travel offer some important parallels to dialysis: minimal space, minimal mobility, and maximal need for comfort. Think of products that would help you weather a long airplane flight. Here are some examples:

- **A moldable neck pillow, such as a "Bucky"**

- **A microwavable neck wrap for warmth**

- **Eye masks, perhaps with lavender scent, for those who sleep during treatments**

- **A lightweight throw; look for a light fleece or faux-cashmere (affordable and washable). The Magellan Catalog for travelers features a throw for airline passengers with a pocket to tuck your feet in for extra warmth, and a zippered pouch for stowing small essentials. And we've seen a great faux cashmere throw at Costco.**

Providing for Thirst and Dryness

- Lemon drops or other hard candy, sugar-free for diabetics

- Lip balm

- Lotion or body butter

- Artificial tears for dry eyes

- Juice boxes

- Water bottles or sports bottles. Many dialysis patients must restrict the amount of fluid they drink. But a small sports bottle—even one designed for a child—would work well. Fill it partially with ice cubes. Martha Stewart would add a slice of lemon or lime; there's no reason we couldn't!

- An insulated beverage container—again, think small volume—for hot beverages like herbal tea.

Providing for Intellectual Stimulation

- Audiobooks

- IPod

- TV, radio and/or laptop

- eBooks/Kindle books (check Amazon.com for something new, maybe something to share)

- Cookbook holder or other gadget to keep a book open to a specific page while you read. Note: depending on fistula placement, it may be difficult for a person to turn pages or operate a laptop easily while on dialysis.

- Adequate light for reading

Providing for Relaxation

- Aromatherapy products like a relaxing essential oil or diffuser

- Music

- Telephone—you will have one anyway for safe dialysis—but also, to keep in touch with the rest of the world

- Crossword puzzles, Sudoku games

- Check with your Home Dialysis patient to see what he/she wants or needs, and build your Comfort Kit accordingly.

Certainly, there are comfort measures for your dialysis patient that cannot be contained in a kit or basket.

Dialysis time is an excellent time to talk with your partner—not about anything that creates tension, of course. But about anything and everything else, including hopes and dreams for the future. He/she could probably use the company; for that matter, so could you!

If your dialysis patient needs foot care, as diabetics do, consider dialysis time for inspecting feet, trimming nails, and giving a relaxing foot massage.

Many people truly hunger for touch—even a brief shoulder rub, a neck scratch. Touch communicates love and acceptance in a way little else can. We think that when a person feels badly because of illness, it is wonderful to experience the positive sensations of their own body! We encourage you to include touch as part of your comfort regimen.

Chapter Sixteen:

Personal Organization: Being an Effective "Bag Lady"

Whether you are the patient or the Home Dialysis helper, effective personal organization will be critical to making your life less stressful and more efficient.

You will find a host of books and other resources on personal organization, and we are not intending to re-invent them. But here are some basic ideas and suggestions that we invite you to consider.

Your life will be more complicated because there is simply more to get done in a day. But it is all doable.

Use a calendar/planner you can carry with you.

A zippered calendar book can be a lifesaver. Beyond your personal schedule, you'll track medical appointments, phone numbers, and ferry or bus schedules. You can even have indexed dividers for kids' school activities, medication lists—anything that fits your life. You can tuck in a skinny calculator, credit card sleeves, and "zip-lock" style plastic envelopes for receipts, stamps, prescriptions. Design it to fit your life.

Simplify whenever and wherever you can.

Except for Home Dialysis treatments, simplify your life by relaxing your standards a little.

- Focus on easy meals, and stock up on healthy snacks you can take for lunch. Buy a Crock Pot. Try some simple recipes. Costco and Trader Joe's have wonderful frozen and pantry items for busy people like us.

- If you are having a family gathering, make it a potluck so everyone can share the work and the cost. Birthday parties can be cake and ice cream only instead of a full meal. And nobody cares—really— if you made anything from scratch.

  (You may care, by the way, and you'll have to come to peace with that. You may truly grieve for days that were more fun. Such grieving is absolutely normal, and we feel that a few visits with a personal counselor should really be included with the package of Home Dialysis!)

- Make clothing and laundry less of a hassle. We don't even bother with clothes that need ironing, and avoid dry cleaning whenever possible. Buy only comfortable clothing you like to wear. We like the kind with forgiving elastic waistbands. Never wear anything that hurts, including shoes.

- Always have a set of underwear and ready-to-wear clothing available to avoid last-minute scrambles.

Remove Clutter!

Clutter fills your mind with extra stress, and you certainly don't need that. Time management experts will advise you to make the bed as soon as you get out of it. One expert says that the whole house revolves around the kitchen sink; if it's clean, the rest of the house will follow. Handle each piece of paper you receive only once. Get rid of your extra paper; give away clothing you can't or won't wear. Clean up kitchen and laundry messes as you go along. Make sure you have laundry hampers and wastebaskets or recycle containers within easy reach—to make it easy to use them.

Get a good tote bag!

A good tote bag is an essential. Here are some tips:

- Find a waterproof, zipper-closed bag, light enough to prevent neck or shoulder pain. Canvas and Goretex are great. We like Land's End and L.L.Bean for practical, lightweight bags (See Appendix 1).

- Get a smaller zippered bag to put inside your tote bag to hold anything that is personally essential, like deodorant, cosmetics, medications, money—things you would need if your plans were suddenly changed. Specifically, if you had to spend the night(s) in the hospital without warning.

- Have a small zippered pouch for credit cards, ID, and enough money for at least a snack, say five dollars.

- Choose attractive—preferably bright—colors for your various pouches. If each pouch is a different color, you can visually identify what you need, and simply grab and go!

- A couple of companies make a removable purse liner with multiple pockets; the idea is to move the liner from bag to bag, making organization easier.

- You will always need a pen and pad of notepaper, so have at least one of each in your tote bag.

- Steve has a personalized L.L.Bean waterproof, zippered tote for all things medical: his medications, dressing supplies, Heart Attack Kit containing nitroglycerine for chest pain. It's the first place we look for medical supplies, and it works well for him.

Figure out a system for your keys!

How frustrating it is to lose your keys, abort an important mission, or just spend extra time because you don't have a good system for keeping track of them. A key leash, a necklace, or a wrist band are simple solutions. And always put the keys down in the same basket, dish, or hang them on the same hook when you get home. Needless to say, planting extra sets in different spots helps, too.

Tuck emergency food in your tote and car.

If you've ever been caught in a hospital after cafeteria hours, you know how valuable a hidden protein bar or other non-perishable food item can be. Juice boxes, cereal bars, individual packs of nuts and fruit can really help in a pinch. Prepaid gift cards (like Starbucks, Subway) are also helpful, and make useful gifts for a family dealing with kidney disease.

Plan ahead for prescription medications for both patient and helper!

Compartmentalized medication boxes can be found in most pharmacies. Twenty-eight-compartment boxes sort and store four doses per day—enough medications for an entire week; these are perfect for patients taking multiple medications. By filling these boxes once a week, you'll stay ahead of the task of ordering important medications.

Don't neglect your personal money management.

With so much going on, it's easy to forget to pay a bill or miss a rent payment or tax deadline. Using your calendar/planner and a Portable Home Office can help keep you out of trouble (see Chapter 17).

Keep gas in the car.

Linda's dad always advised her to fill up with gas when she was down to a quarter of a tank. Don't let forgotten car repairs get you into a bind, either. This may be another stellar example of a project for some loving soul who wants to help you!

Chapter Seventeen:

The Portable Home Office

As we've mentioned before, anything that saves steps saves sanity. We recommend three portable file boxes for the greatest flexibility:

- **A Portable Home Office for mail, bills, and correspondence**
- **A Portable Medical Information File**
- **A Portable Dialysis File: inventory and order sheets, dialysis run logs**

Portable files come in a variety of shapes, sizes, materials, and prices. But you will find a full selection at stores like OfficeMax, Office Depot, or Staples. Stationery and book stores have beautiful items.

> *Use one or more portable files, or all three, as your life requires. The point is to make things easier for you.*

The Portable Home Office

Set up a portable home office so you can tackle chores like sorting mail, paying bills, and doing basic correspondence—anywhere you happen to be.

> *Linda has a portable file box that she can take on the ferry for paying bills while commuting. The same box can be brought to the dialysis room, so she can take care of these chores while Steve is dialyzing.*

Linda's Portable Home Office contains a set of hanging files or file pockets, with labeled dividers including:

- **Incoming mail**
- **Bills to pay**
- **Receipts**
- **"To File"**
- **Individual dividers for each family member**
- **Projects**
- **Miscellaneous**
- **Bill file with alphabetized bills, ready to pay**
- **Check ledger**
- **Stationery and note cards**
- **Stamps**
- **Pens**

The Portable Medical File

Organize your medical papers in a similar way, in a portable file that can travel with you to medical appointments. This might include the following dividers:

- Master list of health care providers' phone numbers, addresses, email

- Business card sheet (clear plastic sheets with multiple openings for business cards. Collect cards from your providers, tuck them into the openings, and place the entire sheet in your file or a 3-ring binder.)

- Medication list

- Lab test results, best filed in chronological order, most recent first

- Diagnostic tests, such as CT scans, ultrasounds

- Hospital/operative records

- Notes taken at doctors' appointments or hospital physician visits

- Instructions, such as pre-operative instructions

- Relevant insurance records

The Portable Dialysis File

Consider building your file with dividers as follows:

- Important phone numbers and contact information for dialysis center

- Dialysis log sheets

- **Supply inventory sheets**

- **Lab requisition sheets**

- **Training materials**

You get the idea: set up portable systems so you can be flexible in keeping up with the work that doesn't stop when dialysis comes home.

Chapter Eighteen:

Traveling With Your Dialysis Machine

Roughly four months into their Home Dialysis experience, Steve and Linda had the opportunity to attend a fitness industry conference in San Diego, California. Since Steve is a consultant to the fitness industry, he would spend hours at the conference: meeting many old friends, exchanging product ideas, and perusing what the competition had to offer. Steve really had to go; it was an industry requirement.

While Steve could have arranged for In-center dialysis in San Diego, he knew he wouldn't have four-hour blocks of time when the convention would be in full swing. And he'd have to be gone for a period of five days, so not dialyzing was not an option.

What to do? Simple—well somewhat simple, anyway. Steve and Linda decided to make the trip, and take Home Hemodialysis on the road. While in San Diego, Steve was able to take full advantage of the convention, and then dialyze in the hotel room during two evenings. It took planning and organization. But they would do it again without hesitation. Here are the tips they took away from their road show:

Planning for the Trip

- Start by learning where the nearest dialysis centers are located in the vicinity of your destination. Keep phone numbers close at hand; you may need assistance, and you won't want to be hunting if you run into difficulties.

- Take your home kidney center contact information with you. You can call long distance; the nurses who trained you have an investment in your faring well on your trip.

- Contact your airline customer service representative directly when you make your flight arrangements. Tell them you will be traveling with a kidney dialysis machine which is critically necessary to sustain your life. Ask your kidney center for a copy of the American Disabilities Act to tuck in your carry-on bag. The ADA protects you from paying extra for the transport of life-sustaining equipment.

- Your kidney center may be able to lend you an aluminum travel box for transporting your dialysis machine. With the machine packed inside, it weighs about one-hundred pounds, and it's bulky—so it goes in the baggage compartment.

- Pre-arrange with your supplier for your dialysate bags to be delivered directly to your hotel. Order several extra bags just in case.

- Find a large zippered duffel bag to hold supplies—and the IV pole from your machine. These will also travel in the baggage compartment.

- Linda found it extremely helpful to pre-package "Ziplock" style gallon bags with the items required for each treatment, such as syringes, four-by-fours, alcohol and iodine wipes, fistula needles or central line caps, whichever

are required. She had an additional bag for general
supplies, such as Heparin, tape, extra gauze pads.

- Lay out the supplies for each individual treatment on
  your bed or kitchen table. Mentally work through each
  step in the process. For each treatment, assemble a
  cartridge, liter of normal saline, warmer disposable,
  waste line, and your pre-packaged daily equipment.
  For each run, include an extra thirty cc syringe; you
  probably won't need it, but you'll have it in case you do.

- In a small tote or other container, place everything
  you would have at the ready at home: your emergency
  directions, Clamp-and-Cut Kit, dialysis manual, logs, and
  flashlight. Don't forget a set or two of IV tubing and an
  extra bag or two of normal saline.

- Consider taking additional full sets of supplies. For
  example, for two planned treatments, we had enough
  supplies for four treatments. Certainly, if you were going
  to do ten treatments on the road, you wouldn't need a
  full twenty sets—but a couple of extra full sets would
  give you some breathing room.

- Pack your critical hemostats—the tiny pliers-like
  instruments that help you loosen connections. (Linda and
  Steve remember their very first run at home: for some
  reason, the hemostats weren't included in their supplies,
  and nobody had noticed! At the end of the run, Linda
  had to unhook Steve from dialysis using a rusty pair of
  household pliers! Not ideal, but time was ticking and Linda
  had to get Steve off the hose before his blood clotted.)

- Pack extra waste lines. You may not be able to reach the
  bathroom or sink from your dialysis location in your
  hotel. Steve and Linda didn't have enough line to reach
  the sink in their beautiful Marriott room overlooking

the bay. So they duct-taped the dialysis waste line
to a waterproof wastebasket which Linda emptied
periodically like an old-fashioned bucket brigade. Steve's
friend, Don Gronachan, who joined in on the maiden
voyage, suggested that Steve simply sling the waste line
over the balcony—an idea that was quickly dismissed.
Remember that you can actually connect two waste lines
together to make a longer line—so be prepared and
pack some extra.

• Take black plastic garbage bags and double-bag dialysis
garbage. Take a small sharps container with you, and
bring your used needles home with you.

• Pack dialysis logs to record your runs on the road.

• Arrange a file folder or envelope to carry the following
paper items:

    • Contact phone numbers for the dialysis center
    nearest your destination, as well as your home
    kidney center, dialysis equipment supplier, and
    24-hour hot lines.

    • Medication list, including list of allergies

    • If possible, include a discharge summary from
    a recent hospital admission. You can get this
    through the Medical Records Department of the
    hospital, at the written request of the patient—
    and can greatly simplify an emergent medical
    evaluation on the road. So can a copy of a recent
    EKG. Linda often gives copies of EKGs taken in
    her office just for this reason.

    • Pack medications in your multiple-compartment
    set, including enough for extra days. Don't forget
    the phosphate binders you take with your meals.

- Carry emergency medications like inhalers, the Heart Attack Kit, or insulin on your person.

Travel Day

- Get plenty of sleep the night before.

- Get up early and allow plenty of time to dissemble and pack your dialysis machine. You would be well advised to give this a practice run.

- Double check your supplies.

- Label your dialysis gear with luggage tags both inside and out!

- You may need help carrying the equipment; it's heavy and bulky.

- Be sure to wear personal ID such as a Medic Alert Tag or identifier from RoadID.com (see Appendix 1).

- Particularly for a longer flight, four hours or more, wear anti-embolism stockings—unless, of course, your personal condition contraindicates these (Try the Magellan Catalog, listed in Appendix 1). Wiggle your toes, move your legs, and get up to stretch during your flight.

- At your hotel, confirm that your dialysis solution has arrived as soon as you check in.

- Once you land in your hotel room, unload and check supplies right away. Don't make the mistake of leaving this until the last minute. You may need to order missing supplies or troubleshoot problems.

During Your Trip

The dialysis patient is well-advised to monitor salt and fluid intake during travel; it's easy to let dietary restrictions slide while on a trip.

Restaurant food is notoriously high in salt, so concentrate on broiled protein, seafood and meat. Request no-salt or low-salt items, and ask for sauces or dressings on the side, if at all.

Other Travel Opportunities

There exists a company which facilitates cruise travel for dialysis patients, who receive dialysis while cruising; dialysis nurses provide the treatments, with nephrologists on board.

We think Home Dialysis could be accomplished with relative ease by a patient and helper on a cruise ship. What a delight it would be to set up equipment and supplies, and have luxury amenities and mobility within the enormous ship! Of course, you'd want to clear this with your cruise line as you make reservations.

Some patients report extended travel via RV. We see the appeal of traveling while the dialysis equipment stays put in one location. And check out Bill Peckham's website for his video clip on his charter boat trip in the Pacific Northwest. (Google up Bill's Blog, "Dialysis From the Sharp End of the Needle.")

Peritoneal Dialysis lends itself easily to travel, because of the lack of a required machine. Stickman Industries offers specific products to facilitate portability of Peritoneal Dialysis.

Steve and Linda enjoy travel, as long as it can be done with relative ease and safety. It does take planning, but you may find that traveling helps you feel more normal and healthy, and more included in the activities of life. Travel allows you to preserve yet another aspect of life that End Stage Renal Disease might otherwise take away!

Chapter Nineteen:

Burnout Ban:
Care for the Caregiver

The Home Dialysis helper is the unsung hero of the whole Home Dialysis operation—particularly with Home Hemodialysis! If you are the helper, you know that the entire operation really does depend on you. We have written this chapter just for you.

Coming to Grips with Some New Realities

You may still be reeling from your partner's diagnosis of kidney failure. Perhaps you had enough warning about the diagnosis of End Stage Renal Disease that you had a chance to talk with other patients, read, and get plenty of information from doctors and dialysis educators beforehand. Perhaps your partner had the opportunity to have a fistula created for dialysis. Or—as in Steve's case—perhaps dialysis started emergently, and things happened so fast that you didn't have any time to process what was really going on.

You may be dealing with some significant mind-occupying fears. You may fear that your partner will become sicker, or die. You may fear being left alone, maybe to raise your children as a single parent.

You may have financial worries or find that private health insurance, Medicare, and social security are a mind-boggling tangle, barely comprehensible at all. You may now be managing on one income, rather than two. And you may have farther-reaching concerns about the adequacy of your savings or life insurance.

You are suddenly dealing with Home Dialysis, which—while a welcome miracle—takes time and effort to absorb. There is an enormous amount to learn—and you will be able to learn it!—but it can be daunting at first. You may feel the weight of the world resting on your shoulders, worried that you won't do the dialysis right, and that something bad will happen as a result.

You may find yourself grieving for days gone by—simpler times when you had none of these worries. You may grieve for lost spontaneity in your life. You may simply grieve for the life you had always imagined. Surely, it didn't include kidney failure and dialysis!

How do you recognize "burnout?"

All caregivers, we believe, experience frustrations and bad days. But sometimes, it goes beyond that—and the caregiver is at risk for burnout. Burnout feels like you can't possibly continue for another day; you're too worn down and bone tired. This can be not only uncomfortable but dangerous for both the helper and the dialysis patient. If our own health suffers, we make more mistakes.

Be on the look-out for the following signs:

- Fatigue

- Irritability, crankiness

- Persistent crying

- Lack of attention to normal grooming and exercise routines (who has time?)

- Lack of attention to the caregiver's own health (Did you omit your mammogram, for example, because your schedule was too busy?)

- Lack of concentration, or difficulty learning things that would normally come easily to you

- Low energy level

- Weight gain or weight loss, without trying

- Lack of interest in usual pleasures

- A feeling that nothing will ever get better

- A feeling of hopelessness or helplessness

- More worry than you would expect, even given your partner's diagnosis

- A sense of hypervigilence: constantly watching for the nuances of your partner's health.

If you've picked up on the fact that most of these signs can be associated with depression, you're right. Burnout and depression may be hard to distinguish. Linda believes that *burnout will generally improve with a good dose of self-care—and continuing to do the things that help.* Depression, on the other hand, lingers on for weeks at a time—not responding as easily to self-care measures and often linked with more serious symptoms such as suicidal thinking.

If you are concerned that you may be depressed, make an appointment to see your primary care provider right away. Depression can be treated in a variety of ways. We think counseling is worth a try. A psychiatrist friend of Linda says, "It's the healthy people who go to therapy!" We think he's right. Exercise also helps. There are also a variety of medications that are well tolerated, and really do work.

Linda tells her patients, "antidepressants don't change the facts of your life. But they can certainly make a difference in how you live your life." Linda's favorite combo in treating her own patients for depression is the triple weapon of counseling, exercise, and antidepressants. It's highly individual, of course. The important thing is to get evaluated, recognize it if you are depressed, and start treatment. By the way, it is also important to understand that antidepressant medications take a few weeks to "take hold," so don't wait until you can barely cope to see your health care provider.

> *Important Warning: If you are feeling so down that you are thinking about suicide, you MUST get help! Call your health care provider. Call the Crisis Clinic, or go directly to a hospital Emergency Room for an evaluation. Things can get better, but only if you're breathing!*

Burnout and "The Giant Breast Syndrome"

Bear with us for a moment if this seems unrelated to Home Dialysis!

When Linda delivered a lot of babies in her practice, she frequently spoke with women about the challenges they experienced when nursing their new babies. Breast feeding, after all, requires two things: nourishment and fluids for the mother to allow her to produce breast milk, and plenty of sucking to stimulate milk production.

Most mothers faced with burnout immediately understand the breast feeding analogy: we all tend to get plenty of sucking—but few of us get enough nourishment! Translated, we all have so many demands on us, we may feel we don't have enough nipples. What we lack is the kind of nourishment required to make more milk.

Another way to look at this is to think of your life energy filling a large bucket. You have plenty of energy, but your bucket has a hole in it! So you have to continually fill your bucket back up, or it will eventually empty completely.

Enough metaphors. Okay, then, let's get down to business. Let's learn how to give ourselves the kind of nourishment that allows us to stay functional and healthy. Here are some approaches that may work for you.

What are your Minimum Daily Requirements?

What do you need every day in the way of food, water, physical exercise, love and affection, intellectual stimulation, and fun? You may not be able to meet every need every day, but you'll stand a better chance—if you start by knowing what you need.

Move your body!

Aerobic exercise, even something as simple as walking, helps to chase burnout away. If possible, start a strength training program, too. This can be done at home. Linda believes the best results for burnout prevention come from vigorous activities that use the body's big muscles. Spinning (cycling) or rowing, for example, burn off calories, frustration, and anger. But these can be logistically challenging. We can all dance to music, and there is a whole industry offering user-friendly exercise videos and DVDs.

Use the HALT acronym

One of Linda's patients shared a great acronym from an Alcoholics Anonymous meeting: "HALT! Don't let yourself get too Hungry, too Angry, too Lonely, or too Tired." Isn't this the essence of self care?

Eat small meals regularly

Many people swear by six "snack meals" per day. Consciously eat fresh, high quality food. Stay away from junk food as much as you can. But if that isn't possible, at least use portion control! Remind yourself that your healthy eating is part of your self-care program to prevent burnout.

Sleep

Good exercise will help you get better sleep, if you're having trouble. Take naps if you can during the day, and on the weekends, allow yourself the opportunity to sleep in if you can.

Take little breaks

Your time is undoubtedly precious. Years ago, a "break" might have been a day or even a week off. Today, you may have a span of only fifteen minutes! Even if you spend the time staring out a window, do it consciously. Actively choose what you do with your time, and appreciate the relief a break provides.

Seek humor

Laughter does help. If you don't come by it naturally, find it in cartoon books, DVDs, or radio shows. There's no shortage; it's a renewable resource, but you may have to look for it.

Listen to music you like

There are no rules here: anything you like will work! Linda used to love spinning classes (indoor cycling) where the instructor featured heavy metal music.

Find creature comforts

You need physical touch, whether that comes in the form of a pedicure, a massage, a spa day, or even the application of lotion. Body butters and scrubs are affordable. Massage training programs offer student massages at a reduced rate; they may not compete with a luxury spa, but who's complaining? Spa certificates, by the way, make wonderful gifts in case someone asks!

Find inexpensive symbolic purchases that say "hang in there!"

Linda recalls another time when her life was in the blender. She started buying earrings. Lots of earrings. Nothing high budget, mind you, but with each earring purchase she reminded herself that she was "on her side." It helped.

Read or Knit

You don't have to finish every novel; this is supposed to be relaxing for you! Do you like to read supermarket magazines? Go for it. If you're a knitter, you may find it a relaxing way to spend your time during treatments. If you are learning, choose simple and quick projects that won't increase your stress level.

Give in, if you need a good cry

Some people have trouble letting go when they're overly stressed. One of Linda's patients rents the DVD Beaches for this purpose. It's a tear-jerker, and she always feels a sense of relief after watching it—and crying—once again.

Stay away from people who sap your energy

We advocate that you surround yourself with as much positivity as you can. If you know people who suck the life out of you, make your contacts brief. By contrast, bring on the people who help to fill up your bucket.

Avoid alcohol and other recreational drugs

Alcohol is a drug, pure and simple. And it works as a depressant. A psychiatrist friend told Linda that it takes only four alcoholic drinks per week to cancel out the effect of an antidepressant for a woman (six per week for a man). Needless to say, other recreational drugs can cloud your mind, cost you money, and steal your precious time.

Negative feelings about your partner are normal—to a point!

Many caregivers report feelings of resentment or negativity about their partners. Linda confides that there have been times when she didn't even like Steve! Talk with your counselor, your health care provider, the social worker at your dialysis center, or other professional if these feelings dominate your thinking. You need a safety valve: release these feelings by talking to someone who can help, but try not to take them out on your partner!

It could be worse

How? Everyday in her medical practice, Linda is reminded that her life could be worse—much worse. Steve and Linda coined a phrase early on in the course of his kidney failure: "It's not the burn unit." It was their shorthand way of acknowledging that they have much to be thankful for.

Give back

Finding small ways to give back to the community grounds you, reminds you that you are not the only one struggling, and helps you remember that help may available to you, too. If you can, buy something for the Food Bank every shopping trip. During the holidays, pick out a gift for one of the charity trees in the mall—in honor of your own struggle, and in gratitude for what you do have. As you prepare for Home Dialysis, you may need to clean out your closets or living space. Give usable clothing and household items to the Goodwill Industries, or other charities. Feeling connected to your community reduces isolation, and helps prevent burnout.

Go to "kidney events"

Participating in the various events sponsored by your local kidney center will help you connect with others who understand, reduce your isolation, and give you practical ideas for coping.

Learn any prayer or meditation that resonates with your heart

Personal favorites here include the Alcoholics Anonymous "Serenity Prayer," and "The Four Agreements."

Accept help from others

Many of us strong, independent types have trouble accepting help from others. We think we can do it all ourselves. Our next chapter is devoted to helping people help you. Read on!

Chapter Twenty:

Helping Others Help You

Have you noticed how often people kindly offer, "Let me know if there's anything I can do to help," or "Call me if I can help in any way"? We think most people really do mean well by this; they really want to help you, but they just don't know what you need. And how could they know? You might not even know what you need!

Our best answer to people who want to help is to have some specific ideas at the ready. We've broken Helping Ideas down into these categories:

- **Help with your physical set-up**
- **Help with preparations for Home Dialysis (not to be confused with helping with the treatments themselves, of course)**
- **Help with food**
- **Help with the home and family**
- **Help with personal support**

Let's explore these, understanding that it can take a village to make all this work. Remember that if you're not specific, you probably won't get what you want. (See Appendix 5 for an exercise to help you identify your needs.)

If you don't have the energy to be direct, show your benevolent friends this chapter! (And if it is simply too much work to delegate, you can always decline offers politely: "I really appreciate your offer; I'll certainly let you know.")

1. Help With Your Physical Set-up

- Moving furniture, equipment and boxes.

- Installing shelving, coat hooks, and hanging pictures.

2. Help With Preparations for Home Dialysis

- Helpers can open, break down, and recycle boxes of dialysis solution.

- Delegate the chore of hanging the dialysate bags— even a break is welcome; remember that you don't want to hang them for hours and hours or they will fall. But certainly twelve hours is okay.

- One of the best tips Linda has found is to pre-pack "Zip-lock" style gallon-sized freezer bags with all the small supplies needed for a single dialysis run. When you are ready for the dialysis run, you just grab a pack and start to work. If you want friends or kids to help assemble these packs, make a detailed, easy-to-read list so they can do it right.

- It is also useful to pre-"pile" each run's stack of cartridges, waste lines, warmer disposables, Chux, and one-liter bags of saline.

- Note: there's no reason why somebody else—even a teenager, for example—can't take over these time-consuming chores. *Every step saved is a step closer to sanity!*

3. Help with food

- While this can be tricky because of special dietary considerations of the dialysis patient, other people in the family need to eat, too. We know it's hard when the dialysis patient is tempted by favorite foods that the rest of the family can eat, but sometimes it is very nice to have something to serve guests or your kids. Cookies, brownies, pumpkin bread are examples of treats that can go in your freezer, but can make your family feel less deprived.

- Prepared meals can be very helpful; sometimes church groups will organize to provide prepared meals for families in a transition. These meals don't have to be homemade.

- Don't forget grocery store gift cards. Think Costco, Trader Joe's, Fred Meyer's/Kroger's—wherever the family typically shops is perfect. And treats like Starbucks cards are wonderful to receive.

- If you're looking for a good food gift for a home with kids, consider sugar-free soft drinks, VitaminWater, or Izzie drinks.

- A practical gift for a family might be a snack gift pack: microwave popcorn, fruit leather, cereal, individual packs of chips, or crackers—particularly things that might not be affordable in the family's food budget!

4. Help with Home and Family

• Steve's niece, Deanna, stepped up to provide housecleaning services for a period of several months. What a gift! A gift certificate to a housecleaning agency for even a one-time cleaning would be exceptional as well. But remember that some people have very personal feelings about having others see the details of their lives; check first to make sure this gift would be welcome. Linda's mom, for example, says she'd work to clean up before a housekeeper came—not the perfect gift for her, we imagine.

• Shopping help, like a Costco run, is a kind gesture.

• Yard help, runs to the garbage dump, changing high-ceiling light bulbs are all enormously helpful.

• Childcare may allow for a couple's evening out.

• Movie tickets (gift certificates), restaurant gift certificates, a NetFlix gift card are good entertainment ideas.

• Since many families on dialysis are financially strapped, think of extras that a family might not put on their own budget, like concert tickets, day camp scholarships, lessons for the kids. We already feel a bit inadequate in the parenting department when our energies are stretched so thin; extras that add quality to kids' lives help parents feel more capable!

• Providing rides for a patient can be invaluable. Linda's Office Manager, Barb, chipped in to pick up Linda's mom from her hair appointments—a task that was critical to Mom, but didn't always mesh with Steve's doctors' appointments.

5. Help with Personal Support

- Almost anything is helpful and appreciated—as long as it doesn't create extra work for the recipient in orchestrating the details of the help!

- What is the thing the caregiver would never lavish on themselves. Give that.

- Pedicure certificates, spa certificates can provide brief, needed getaways.

- Linda's mom used to send a card every Thanksgiving that included stamps and a coffee gift card.

You get the idea: people want to help! And you can help them be better helpers, for the benefit of all concerned.

If you are one of the many people who has difficulty accepting help, remember that giving can be invaluable to the giver as well as the recipient. Remember, it's not all about you! Let others rise to the occasion and participate, too.

Chapter Twenty-One:

Reclaiming Your Bedroom and Bath

We realize that many people do overnight Home Dialysis runs in bed, and these extended runs are favored by many dialysis patients. If you are performing shorter runs, however, we encourage you to do them somewhere besides the bedroom.

Here's why we make that recommendation. When your life is necessarily focused on illness and the very critical realities of Home Dialysis, we believe you need a place of peace and privacy. You need a place where at the end of a busy day, you can simply let down and let go of your tensions and worries.

You need a place where the lights can be dimmed, where you can read, or talk, or just relax together.

You need a place where you can cuddle, where you can share the simple comfort of holding each other. Whether it's sexual or not, it is intimate—and necessary. All humans need the comfort of touch. When a person is feeling ill much of the time, the pleasure of positive sensations from one's own body remind us that we are alive. Backrubs, body brushing, getting a good back scratch or massage with lotion may be the most positive physical experiences your patient feels.

Needless to say, it communicates love and belonging—for both of you.

Preserving the sanctity of your bedroom allows you to feel more adult, more participatory, and less dependent. It helps nurture you as a couple. Keeping your bedroom as your private retreat, you make a statement that your relationship is important—something to be protected.

If you are fortunate enough to have a bathroom for the two of you, the same recommendation applies. Resist the practical temptation to make it into an extension of a sickroom. Keep it clean, private, and comfortable. If you have medical equipment, bandage and dressing supplies, or medications which must live in your bathroom, use Jane's pointers in finding attractive baskets to camouflage these items while still keeping them accessible.

You have made many compromises and sacrifices because of kidney disease. Think carefully about how you can achieve as much normalcy as possible while still respecting the realities of your life.

CONCLUSION:

Going Forward

In *Arranging Your Life When Dialysis Comes Home*, we have intro-
duced you to the world of Home Dialysis: a world you may already
know, or an unfamiliar no-man's land you've just learned you need
to travel. We have told you our stories so you'll know that we truly
understand how impactful kidney disease and Home Dialysis can
be on a couple, a family, and on a home.

Home Dialysis is a true miracle with many challenges. We've of-
fered advice on planning ahead but we understand that many of us
will have to backtrack—to go back to square one to really reclaim
our homes.

We've shown you the option of Home Dialysis but we've also
been blunt about the reasons it's not always easy. But support is
there, with knowledgeable twenty-four hour "hotline" nurses and
technicians available to help you. There's an excellent foundation of
Home Dialysis Training—complete with caring nurses who recognize that Home Dialysis can really make your life more livable.

Our crash course in design can help you see possibilities for your
own Home Dialysis Center. We have discussed workable storage
solutions, room layout, and organizational tips. We have made

special efforts to keep suggestions affordable, practical, and easy to execute.

Finally, we focused on helping you organize the details of your life to make it more manageable. We looked carefully at the role of the caregiver, with particular attention to the concept of caregiver burnout and how it can be prevented. We've encouraged allowing others to help and given you specific ideas on what to ask for.

We know there will be many more people on dialysis in the future as our Baby Boom generation moves further into mid-life. Sadly, many Americans will experience lifestyle-related kidney failure which might have been prevented. We hope our next generation will learn from our experiences and take steps to prevent kidney disease.

There is no cure today for End Stage Renal Disease—and nothing trumps healthy kidneys, but we see hope on the horizon for easier, more effective dialysis options. We also see enormous promise in the gift of kidney transplantation and great hope in efforts to make transplantable kidneys available to more people.

In the meantime, we hope we've made a small contribution in the area of improving the quality of life for people with renal failure. If even one pointer or suggestion in our book provides a little help or relief, we will count ourselves successful.

We wish you the very best in your personal journey. May you live long and healthfully, and *in the comfort of your underwear!*

Visit Linda Gromko, MD and Designer Jane McClure on our website at www.Arrange2Live.com for ongoing information, helpful products, and new ideas.

We also welcome your personal stories and ideas. Please give us your feedback to better enable us to help others along this road.

CONTACT US AT:
www.Arrange2Live.com

MAILING ADDRESS:
Arrange2Live
16025 11th Avenue NE
Seattle, Washington 98155

APPENDIX ONE

Products and Resources We Like

Furnishings and Furniture:

IKEA—Pax wardrobe systems in 24"depths for dialysis solution storage (When possible, use the taller cabinet heights to maximize storage options.); Kitchen, entertainment and office cabinet options used in conjunction with wardrobes to provide a consistent look; Many textile and accessory offerings at reasonable price ranges and excellent quality.

PierOne—Import store with great baskets, accessories.

CostPlus—Import store with great baskets, accessories.

Costco, Sam's Club—Hard to beat warehouse stores for small furnishings, storage, office supplies.

Bed, Bath, and Beyond—Storage, Textiles, small furnishings.

Draperies:

IKEA—Look to IKEA for extra-long panels; helpful catalog.

JC Penney Company—On-line catalog—and some retail outlets—can be excellent resources.

Google On-line resource:—enter "extra-long or extra-wide drapery panels;" also Google up "screens."

KS Systems—Hardware for hanging draperies from ceilings—available only through interior designer.

Bed, Bath, and Beyond—Drapery panels at reasonable cost; on-line purchases available.

Lighting:

Lamps Plus, IKEA—Affordable assortment of different styles, uplighting, accent and task lighting.

Office Supplies:

Office Depot, Office Max, Staples, Costco, Sam's Club—Standard supplies; great for portable office accessories.

Totes and luggage:

LL Bean; Land's End—Waterproof canvas or Gore-tex bags with zippers and generous sizes.

Personal Comfort:

Bucky—Moldable neck and arm pillows.

Bath and Body Works—Affordable lotions, scrubs, and candles.

Magellan Travel Catalog—Items designed for travel but ideal for those who must spend hours in a dialysis chair.

Pier One; CostPlus—Excellent assortment of candles.

Travel Products:

Magellan Travel Catalog—Personal comfort products adaptable for dialysis.

MedicAlert; RoadID.com—Personal identification to wear

Intellectual Stimulation/Entertainment:

Amazon.com—Kindle (new electronic book product that requires one hand for turning pages).

Netflix—Mail delivery of DVDs.

Paint:

Benjamin Moore—Low VOC latex interior paint in matte finish.

Furniture Consignment:

In Seattle, Consign Design and Armadillo Consignment. Elsewhere, look on-line for "Furniture Consignment."

Salvage:

In Seattle, The REStore for architectural salvage for building materials "with a past;" Earthwise for recycled architectural salvage, cabinets, and the like. Elsewhere, look On-line for "salvage."

Thriftshops:

Goodwill Industries, Salvation Army, Value Village, Hospital Thriftshops, St. Vincent De Paul.

Discount Stores:

Target, Fred Meyer, Target, TJ Maxx, Marshalls, Costco, Sam's Club.

Medical Supplies:

Costco, Sam's Club, Stickman Industries (for Peritoneal Dialysis supplies), and—selectively—eBay!

APPENDIX TWO:

Traceable Furniture and Room Sketch Page
& Graph Paper

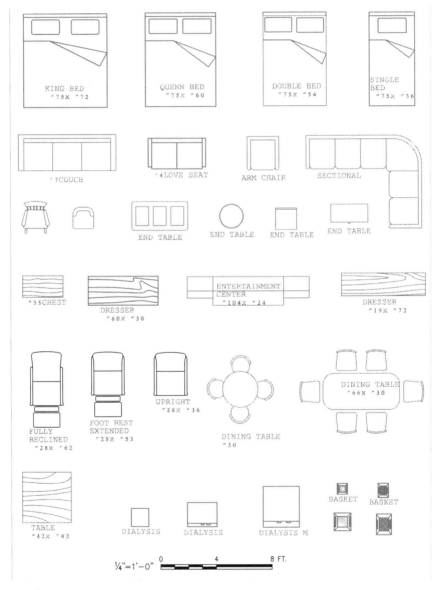

KING BED
"75X "72

QUENN BED
"75X "60

DOUBLE BED
"75X "54

SINGLE BED
"75X "36

'7COUCH

'4LOVE SEAT

ARM CHAIR

SECTIONAL

END TABLE

END TABLE

END TABLE

END TABLE

"35CHEST

DRESSER
"60X "30

ENTERTAINMENT CENTER
"104X "24

DRESSER
"19X "72

UPRIGHT
"28X "36

FULLY RECLINED
"28X "62

FOOT REST EXTENDED
"28X "53

DINING TABLE
"30

DINING TABLE
"66X "30

TABLE
"42X "42

DIALYSIS

DIALYSIS

DIALYSIS M

BASKET

BASKET

¼"=1'-0" 0 4 8 FT.

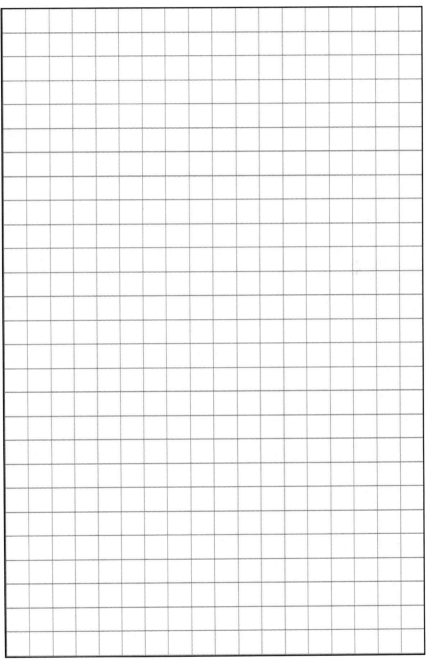

¼"=1'-0" 0   4   8 FT.

APPENDIX THREE:

Waste Line Pass-Through Example

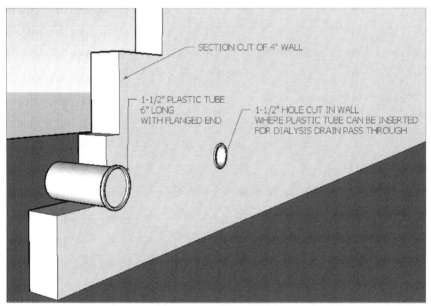

Note: the 'hole' at the left of the diagram shows the Pass-Through in cross-section. The 'hole' at the right illustrates the finished product. Remember not to attempt this project if you do not have the appropriate skill set!

APPENDIX FOUR:

Jane's Storage Wall Based on IKEA Cabinets

IKEA product names and measurements used to construct the west wall storage configuration in the Guest Room Makeover.

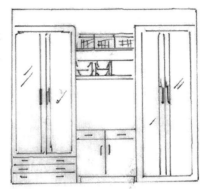

1 **Pax wardrobe** 39⅜" x 23⅜" x 92⅞" H (These wardrobes come in two different heights. Make sure to check your ceiling measurement to order the correct height for your room.)

1 **Pax Ballstad wardrobe** with drawers

1 **Akurum base cabinet** w/2 drawers/36" w x 24⅛" d x 30" h

1 **Countertop**/birch cut-to-size

1 **Barnslig** wall storage unit (from children's section) 36" w.

2 **Broder shelves** 46⅞" l (cut-to-size)

Pax shelves: 5 shelves for right-hand cabinet

    7 shelves for the left-hand cabinet

3 **Flort storage boxes** w/lids

(All items listed above sourced from the 2009 IKEA catalog.)

APPENDIX FIVE:

"Asking for Help" Exercise

Serving as the helper for a Home Dialysis patient requires considerable time and energy. Yet caregivers sometimes find it difficult to ask for help.

Before you can get the most effective help, it's best to know what it is that you need. Identify your own needs in the following categories. Feel free to add your own categories as well.

I could use help in:

- ☐ Preparing my home for Home Dialysis.
- ☐ Taking care of others who depend on me besides the kidney patient, such as kids or parents.
- ☐ Shopping for food.
- ☐ Preparing meals, maybe even cooking ahead for future meals.
- ☐ Organizing medical supplies and medications.
- ☐ Transportation: rides and car maintenance.
- ☐ Meeting my own personal needs (exercise, social, medical, personal care).
- ☐ Managing money, paying bills, doing financial planning.
- ☐ Doing chores around the house.
- ☐ Providing treats for my family: things I used to provide.

☐ Getting ready for holidays or special occasions.

☐ Housecleaning and home maintenance.

☐ Other:

_____

_____

_____

_____

_____

If my best friend were in my exact situation, here's what I would do for her/him:

_____

_____

_____

_____

_____

_____

_____

_____

_____

_____

Color Palette Suggestions

Basic Color	Hue Options	Ben Moore Color Ideas
Purple	Eggplant, dusty lavenders, violets, indigo	2113-40 Cinnamon Slate, 2115-40 Mauve Blush, 2114-50 Victorian Mauve
Reds	Terra cotta, russet, spice, clay, blush	2166-40 Soft Pumpkin, AC-50 Colorado Clay, 2090-30 Terra Cotta Tile
Beige	Sand, tan, taupe, wheat	2151-60 Linen Sand, HC-23 Yorkshire Tan, HC-43 Tyler Taupe
Green	Sage, pear, apple, moss, lichen	2144-30 Rosemary Sprig, 2145-40 Fernwood Green, 2145-50 Limesickle
Blue	Silvers, gray, mist, haze	HC-156 Van Deusen Blue, 2123-30 Sea Star, 2136-60 Harbor Haze
Yellow	Butter, cream, gold ivory, honey	2151-50 Bronzed Beige, HC-31 Waterbury Cream, HC-17 Summerdale Gold
Neutrals	Gray, tan, taupe, whites, black, browns	HC-78 Litchfield Gray, AC 33-Mesa Verde Tan, AC 32-Pismo Dunes

Made in the USA
San Bernardino, CA
13 February 2016